MANAGEMENT

OF

HYPERTENSION

Eighth Edition

by Norman M. Kaplan, MD

Department of Internal Medicine
The University of Texas
Southwestern Medical School
5323 Harry Hines Boulevard
Dallas, Texas 75235-8899

 medical publishers

Direct Mail Orders
EMIS, Inc.
P.O. Box 820062
Dallas, TX 75382-0062

Telephone Orders
1-800-225-0694

FAX Your Order
(214) 349-2266
http:\\www.emispub.com

Management of Hypertension
Eighth Edition

ISBN: 0-917634-10-1

Published in the United States 2002

Printed in the United States of America

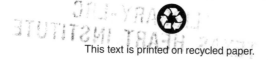

This text is printed on recycled paper.

TABLE OF CONTENTS

FIGURES

TABLES

FOREWORD

This book should be useful to those who want a ready, up-to-date reference to practical issues in the treatment of hypertensive patients. My larger book, *Kaplan's Clinical Hypertension,* now in its eighth edition, provides additional background, details, and references for those who need them.

I am pleased that both books have been so well received as to warrant eight editions. This latest one has been extensively revised to keep it as current as modern publishing can. In addition, this handbook has been structured to provide specific guidelines for the management of various prototypes, e.g., the elderly, diabetic, dyslipidemics, patients with coronary disease, and many of the other conditions that commonly coexist with hypertension.

This book may be provided free to the reader by a pharmaceutical company. That arrangement has been handled by the publisher without the author's knowledge of which company would do so. Nothing in the text is intended to favor any product in a manner beyond the scientific evidence known to the author.

I thank all my coworkers, both in Dallas and elsewhere, who have provided me with the data and insights needed to write this book.

Norman M. Kaplan, M.D.

#1 Measurement of Blood Pressure

General Principles

The first and most important step in the management of hypertension is a careful assessment of the level of the blood pressure (BP). BPs must be taken frequently and carefully. The BP naturally varies a great deal, so it is important to avoid all controllable causes of variation. During 24-hour ambulatory monitoring, pressures while awake may vary by more than 30 mm Hg, mostly in association with physical and emotional stresses.

Much lower levels are usual during sleeping, with the important exception of higher readings during periods of sleep apnea. A marked rise in pressure occurs upon rising from bed, contributing to the increased incidence of cardiovascular catastrophes in the early morning hours.

In order to avoid the alerting reaction that is responsible for the white-coat effect—an often significant rise in BP when taken in an office setting, more so than if taken by physicians than nurses—readings should be taken out of the office. Ambulatory monitoring is easiest but too expensive for routine use. For most, home recording is satisfactory, using inexpensive but accurate electronic devices that automatically record the pressure (e.g., Omron HEM-7226, available for $40).

Establishing the Diagnosis

For those unable to obtain out-of-the-office readings, at least three sets of three readings should be taken with intervals of two weeks or more between sets unless the initial levels are so high (BPs above 180/100 mm Hg) or target-organ damage is so ominous as to demand immediate intervention. Levels of BP tend to fall after the first set of readings, with most of the fall noted during the first few weeks.

Although higher office readings may indicate higher risks for the subsequent development of cardiovascular disease (CVD), the average of multiple out-of-the-office readings taken over one or two months should be taken to establish the diagnosis of hypertension and to decide upon the need for therapy. Home readings average 5 to 10 mm Hg lower than office readings.

Monitoring Progress of Therapy

Only occasional follow-up office readings are needed. To ensure adequate control by antihypertensive therapy, readings should be taken at the end of a dosing interval. Once the goal of therapy is reached and the patient is asymptomatic, office readings need only be obtained every four to six months.

For others, more frequent readings taken out of the office will be useful. These include patients with:

- Poor control based on office blood pressure, despite increased medication.
- Advancing target-organ damage, despite apparent good control based on office readings.
- Symptoms that could reflect hypotension.

Home readings are helpful to ensure 24-hour control of hypertension, with a particular need to document that the early morning surge in pressure is moderated in hopes of avoiding the high incidence of cardiovascular catastrophes between 6:00 and 10:00 a.m.

FIGURE 1.1

Taking the Blood Pressure

1. The patient should be relaxed and the arm must be supported. Ensure no tight clothing constricts the arm.

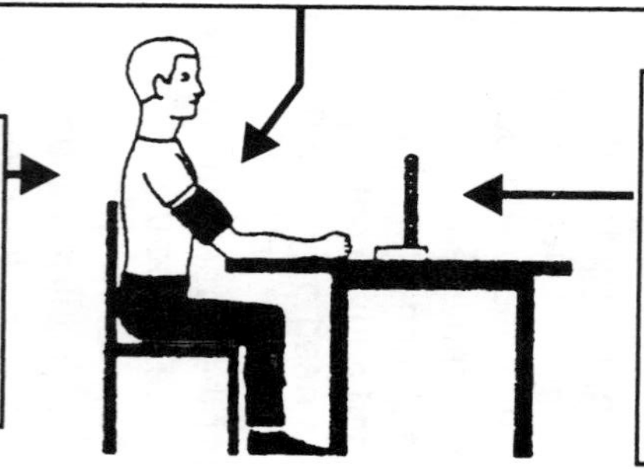

2. The cuff must be level with the heart. If arm circumference exceeds 33 cm, a large cuff must be used. Place stethescope diaphragm over brachial artery.

3. The column of mercury must be vertical. Inflate to occlude the pulse. Deflate at 2 to 3 mm Hg per heartbeat. Measure systolic (first sound) and diastolic (cessation of sound) to nearest 2 mm Hg.

Technique for measurement of blood pressure recommended by the British Hypertension Society (From J Hypertens 1985;3:293).

TABLE 1.1

Guidelines for Measurement of Blood Pressure

Defining Factors	Response
Patient Conditions	
Posture	Initially, particularly >65 years, with diabetes, or receiving antihypertensive therapy, check for postural changes by taking readings after 5 min supine, then immediately upon and 2 min after standing.
	For routine follow-up, the patient should sit quietly for 5 min with the arm bared and supported at the level of the heart and the back resting against a chair.
Circumstances	No caffeine or smoking within 30 min preceding the reading.
	No exogenous adrenergic stimulants (e.g., phenylephrine in nasal decongestants).
	A quiet, warm setting.
Equipment	
Cuff Size	Since a too-small bladder may cause falsely high readings, the bladder should encircle at least 80% of the circumference and cover two-thirds of the length of the arm.
Manometer	Either a mercury, recently calibrated aneroid or validated electronic device.
For Infants	Use ultrasound (e.g., the Doppler method).
Technique	
Number of Readings	On each occasion, take at least two readings, separated by as much time as is practical; if readings vary >5 mm Hg, take additional readings until two are close.

Guidelines for Measurement of Blood Pressure

Defining Factors	Response

Technique (continued)

Number of Readings	For diagnosis, obtain three sets of readings at least one week apart.
	Initially, take pressure in both arms; if the pressures differ, use the arm with the higher pressure.
	If the arm pressure is elevated, take the pressure in one leg, particularly in patients <30 years old.
Performance	Inflate the bladder quickly to a pressure 20 mm Hg above the systolic pressure, recognized by disappearance of radial pulse, to avoid an auscultatory gap.
	Deflate the bladder 3 mm Hg/heartbeat.
	Record the Korotkoff phase I (appearance) and phase V (disappearance).
	If the Korotkoff sounds are weak, have the patient raise the arm and open and close the hand 5-10 times, then inflate the bladder quickly.
Recordings	Note the pressure, patient position, the arm, and cuff size (e.g., 140/90, seated, right arm, large adult cuff).

References

American Society of Hypertension: Recommendations for routine blood pressure measurement by indirect cuff sphygmomanometry. *Am J Hypertens* 1992;5:207–209.

Beevers G, Lip GYH, O'Brien E. Blood pressure measurement. Part I—Sphygmomanometry: Factors common to all techniques. *Br Med J* 2001a;322:981–985.

Beevers G, Lip GYH, O'Brien E. Blood pressure measurement. Part II—Conventional sphygmomanometry: Technique of auscultatory blood pressure measurement. *Br Med J* 2001b;322:1043–1046.

Gosse P, Cipriano C, Bemurat L, et al.: Prognostic significance of blood pressure measured on rising. *J Hum Hypertens* 2001;15:413–417.

Johnstone MT, Mittleman M, Tofler G, Muller JE: The pathophysiology of the onset of morning cardiovascular events. *Am J. Hypertens* 1996;9:22S–28S.

Marcia G, et al.: Alerting reaction and rise in blood pressure during measurement by physician and nurse. *Hypertension* 1987;9:209–215.

O'Brien E, Beevers G, Lip GYH: Blood pressure measurement. Part III—Automated sphygmomanometry: Ambulatory blood pressure measurement. *Br Med J* 2001a;322:1110–1114.

O'Brien E, Waeber B, Parati G, et al.: Blood pressure measuring devices: Recommendations of the European Society of Hypertension. *Br Med J* 2001b;322:531–536.

Pickering T, Kaplan NM, Krakoff L, et al.: Recommendations for the use of home (self) and ambulatory blood pressure monitoring. *Am J Hypertens* 1995;9:1–11.

Reeves RA: Does this patient have hypertension? How to measure blood pressure. *JAMA* 1995;273:1211–1218.

Rogers MAM, Small D, Buchan DA, et al.: Home monitoring service improves mean arterial pressure in patients with essential hypertension. *Ann Intern Med* 2001;134:1024–1032.

#2 Definition of Hypertension

2.

General Definition

Based on the relative increase in risks, hypertension may be defined as sustained average levels of systolic blood pressure (SBP) above 140 mm Hg and/or diastolic blood pressure (DBP) levels above 90 mm Hg in adult patients. The presence of DBP below 90 but SBP above 140 is defined as isolated systolic hypertension (ISH). These levels have been proposed as the upper limit of normal for children in the 50th percentile in height:

Age (years)	Blood Pressure (mm Hg)	
	Girls	*Boys*
1	104/58	102/57
6	111/73	114/74
12	123/80	126/82
17	129/84	134/85

In patients under age 50, hypertension is usually manifested by rises in both systolic and diastolic levels. However, as patients age, atherosclerotic rigidity or stiffness of the large arteries usually causes the systolic levels to rise, whereas diastolic levels tend to fall. In patients over age 60, ISH is the most common form of hypertension. Since both the rising systolic and falling diastolic levels reflect atherosclerosis, it is not surprising that the difference between the two—the pulse pressure—is most closely correlated with the risk for cardiovascular events since they too are predominantly secondary to atherosclerosis.

Classification by Degree

The 1997 Joint National Committee (JNC) report classified the degree of hypertension thusly:

Category	Systolic (mm Hg)	Diastolic (mm Hg)
Normal	<130	<85
High-Normal	130 to 139	85 to 89
Hypertension:		
Stage 1	140 to 159	90 to 99
Stage 2	160 to 179	100 to 109
Stage 3	≥180	≥110

The relative frequency of various levels of diastolic hypertension in a large population of people screened at home by the Hypertension Detection and Follow-up Program was about 70% between 90 and 99 mm Hg, 20% between 100 and 109 mm Hg, and 10% above 110 mm Hg (see Figure 2.1).

Those patients with DBPs from 85 to 89 mm Hg may be classified as high-normal. They should be rechecked more frequently and counseled more vigorously to follow the nondrug modalities (see Section #9 and #10) that may decrease the likelihood of progression of hypertension while improving overall cardiovascular status at little financial cost or interference with the quality of life. Cessation of smoking will not only lower BP but is the single most beneficial move to improve cardiovascular health.

Operational Definition

Caution is needed in having enough BP measurements under appropriate conditions before making the diagnosis of hypertension. Logically, the label should be affixed only if active therapy is indicated. People labeled as hypertensive may suffer from increased psychoneurotic and other complaints, resulting in an increase in absenteeism from work. In addition, the label may be responsible for added economic burdens, e.g., higher life insurance premiums and loss of job opportunities.

There is, then, a need to balance the risks of not diagnosing and treating a level of BP against the costs and risks of doing so. In addition to costs of labeling, there are potential side effects from all currently used antihypertensive drugs.

As noted in Section #11, more than the BP level should be considered in deciding on appropriate management. Some patients with BP levels above 140/90 mm Hg may not require immediate antihypertensive drug therapy, whereas some at high overall cardiovascular risk should be treated with medications even with BPs below 140/90 mm Hg.

White-Coat Hypertension

About 20% of patients with BPs that are persistently above 140/90 mm Hg in the physician's office have average daytime levels by either ambulatory monitoring or multiple self-recorded readings that are below 130/80. Such "white-coat" or "isolated office" hypertension is noted more frequently in patients with office readings below 160/100, women, elderly, nonsmokers, and in the absence of left ventricular hypertrophy. In most follow-up studies for as long as 10 years, these patients develop little more CVD than persistently normotensive subjects. Longer follow-up may reveal more danger, so such patients obviously should be closely monitored and strongly advised to improve unhealthy lifestyles.

Exercise Hypertension

Patients who are normotensive at rest but whose SBP rises above 200 mm Hg during exercise stress tests have a greater likelihood of developing persistent hypertension. Nonetheless, the majority remain normotensive so that they should not be labeled as "prehypertensive." As with white-coat hypertensives, they should be more carefully monitored and advised to follow healthy lifestyles, in particular, regular aerobic exercise to modulate their response to physical stress.

FIGURE 2.1

The Distribution of Levels of Diastolic Blood Pressure

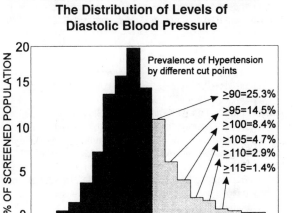

Prevalence of Hypertension by different cut points

$\geq$90=25.3%
$\geq$95=14.5%
$\geq$100=8.4%
$\geq$105=4.7%
$\geq$110=2.9%
$\geq$115=1.4%

Frequency distribution of diastolic blood pressure at home screen (158,906 persons ages 30 to 69). (From The Hypertension Detection and Follow-Up Program. Circulation Research 40 (Suppl 1):106, 1977, by permission of the American Heart Association, Inc.)

References

Burt VL, Whelton P, Roccella EJ, et al.: Prevalence of hypertension in the U.S. adult population. *Hypertension* 1995;25: 305–313.

Franklin SS, Jacobs MJ, Wong ND, et al.: Predominance of isolated systolic hypertension among middle-aged and elderly US hypertensive. *Hypertension* 2001;37:869–874.

Joint National Committee. The sixth report of the Joint National Committee on Detection, Evaluation, and Treatment of High Blood Pressure. *Arch Intern Med* 1997;157:2413–2446.

Kannel WB: Blood pressure as a cardiovascular risk factor: Prevention and treatment. *JAMA* 1996;275:1571–1576.

Laurent S, Boutouyrie P, Asmar R, et al.: Aortic stiffness is an independent predictor of all-cause and cardiovascular mortality in hypertensive patients. *Hypertension* 2001;37:1236–1241.

MacDonald LA, Sackett DL, Haynes RB, Taylor DW: Labeling in hypertension: A review of the behavioral and psychological consequences. *J Chronic Dis* 1984;37:933–942.

MacMahon S, Peto R, Cutler J, et al.: Blood pressure, stroke, and coronary heart disease, Part 2: Prolonged differences in blood pressure: Prospective observational studies corrected for the regression dilution bias. *Lancet* 1990;335:765–774.

NHBPEP Working Group: Update of the 1987 task force report on high blood pressure in children and adolescents. *Pediatrics* 1996;98:649–658.

Prospective Studies Collaboration: Cholesterol, diastolic blood pressure, and stroke: 13,000 strokes in 450,000 people in 45 prospective cohorts. *Lancet* 1995;346:1647–1653.

Sharabi Y, Ben-Cnaan R, Hanin A, et al. The significance of hypertensive response to exercise as a predictor of hypertension and cardiovascular disease. *J Hum Hypertens* 2001;15: 353–356.

Verdecchia P, Palatini P, Schillaci G, et al.: Independent predictors of isolated systolic ('white-coat') hypertension. *J Hypertens* 2001a;19:1015–1020.

Verdecchia P, Schillaci G, Reboldi G, et al.: Different prognostic impact of 24-hour mean blood pressure and pulse pressure on stroke and coronary artery disease in essential hypertension. *Circulation* 2001b;103:2579–2584.

Whelton PK: Epidemiology of hypertension. *Lancet* 1994;344: 101–106.

#3 Types of Hypertension

Primary Hypertension
Secondary Hypertension
Special Populations

3.

PRIMARY HYPERTENSION

In typical clinical practice, 95% of hypertensive adults ages 18 to 65 will have no identifiable cause; thus, their hypertension should be defined as primary, essential, or idiopathic.

SECONDARY HYPERTENSION

The frequency of secondary forms of hypertension will likely approximate:
- Renal parenchymal disease—3–4%
- Renal vascular hypertension—0.5–1%
- Adrenal hyperfunction—0.1–0.3%, to include:
  - Pheochromocytoma
  - Cushing's syndrome
  - Primary aldosteronism
- Miscellaneous causes—0.1–0.3%

As will be noted in Section #6, claims for a much higher prevalence of primary aldosteronism have recently been published.

SPECIAL POPULATIONS

Populations composed of varying proportions of special groups of patients will have different frequencies than those listed above.

Adults with Severe or Resistant Hypertension

Patients with accelerated (Grade 3 fundi) or malignant (Grade 4 fundi) hypertension or whose hypertension remains resistant to appropriate therapy have higher frequencies of renal parenchymal disease and, even more so, of renal vascular hypertension (RVH). The frequency of renal vascular hypertension may be as high as 33% in such patients (see Section #5).

Women Taking Oral Contraceptives

After starting estrogen-containing oral contraceptives (OCs), most women experience a 2 to 4 mm Hg increase in BP. As many as 5% of previously normotensive women will have a rise in DBP above 90 mm Hg after five years of pill use, a rate two to three times higher than women not taking the pill. The reason BP rises more in some women is unknown, but these women may have a pre-existing propensity to develop primary hypertension or an underlying renal dysfunction (see Section #7).

Children

Prepubertal hypertensive children most likely have a renal cause. Postpubertal children most likely have primary hypertension, but a higher frequency of secondary causes is seen among them (see Section #30).

Elderly

Patients who have onset of hypertension after age 50, and even more so after age 60, have a higher frequency of renal parenchymal disease and RVH.

References

Anderson GH Jr, Blakeman N, Streeten DHP: The effect of age on prevalence of secondary forms of hypertension in 4,429 consecutively referred patients. *J Hypertens* 1994;12: 609–615.

August P, Praril S: Hypertension in women. *J Clin Endocrinol Metab* 1999;84:1862.

Bartosh SM, Aronson AJ: Childhood hypertension. *Pediatr Clin North Am* 1999;46:235–252.

Burt VL, Cutler JA, Higgins M, et al.: Trends in the prevalence, awareness, treatment, and control of hypertension in the adult U.S. population. *Hypertension* 1995;26:60–69.

Hannaford PC, Croft PR, Kay CR: Oral contraception and stroke. *Stroke* 1994;25:935–942.

Safian RD, Textor SC: Renal-artery stenosis. *N Engl J Med* 2001;344:431–442.

NOTES

#4 Primary Hypertension

Background

The specific cause of primary hypertension is unknown (Figure 4.1). A genetic predisposition has been documented, with about a twofold higher incidence in those with a close relative who is hypertensive. Environmental factors that increase the incidence include:

- Obesity, particularly upper body
- Psychogenic stress
- High sodium intake
- Alcohol intake greater than one ounce per day

Low birth weight from intrauterine growth retardation may be an important precursor of adult hypertension. The problem may be most important in populations with repeated pregnancies in immature women who receive inadequate diets and healthcare.

BPs may rise as a consequence of an increase in either cardiac output or peripheral resistance (see Figure 4.2). Although cardiac output may be high initially, hypertension usually persists because of increased peripheral resistance. This, in turn, may arise from both functional tightening and structural thickening of resistance vessels. Multiple factors may be responsible. Resistance to the actions of insulin in peripheral muscles has been shown in hypertensives, and the resultant hyperinsulinemia may serve as a stimulus for hypertension. Insulin resistance may be part of the "metabolic syndrome" of glucose intolerance/diabetes, dyslipidemia, and microalbuminuria. A host of other pressor and hypertrophic factors have been discovered; endothelium-derived relaxing factor (nitric oxide) and endothelin are two that likely are involved in human hypertension.

The disease usually:

- Appears between ages 30 and 50
- Is slowly progressive
- Remains asymptomatic until significant target-organ damage appears after 10 to 20 years. Early symptoms may reflect anxiety-induced hyperventilation.

Evaluation

A complete history and pertinent physical examination should be followed by a limited laboratory evaluation to:

- Assess target-organ damage
- Rule out secondary causes
- Ascertain overall cardiovascular risk

The laboratory evaluation includes:

- Hematocrit
- Urine analysis
- Automated blood chemistries, including:
  - Creatinine
  - Fasting glucose
  - Sodium
  - Potassium
  - Total cholesterol
  - HDL-cholesterol
- Electrocardiogram

Additional tests may be needed for those in the previously noted special populations or who display suggestive features of a secondary cause by history or physical examination (see Table 4.1). (Details of these tests are provided in their respective sections of this text.)

In the future, additional procedures may be more frequently indicated as more sensitive indices of the severity of hypertension are developed. These procedures include:

- Echocardiography, which shows left ventricular hypertrophy much earlier than electrocardiography
- 24-hour ambulatory BP monitoring, which has been found to predict the development of target-organ damage more accurately than office measurements
- Assay for urinary microalbuminuria
- Measures of arterial compliance

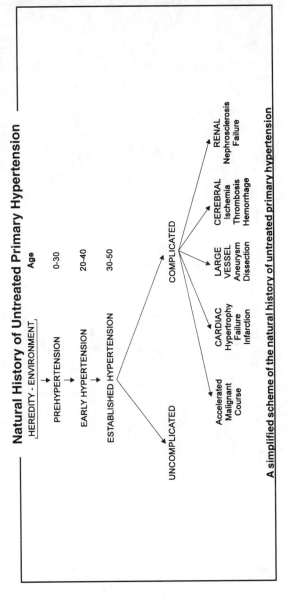

Natural History of Untreated Primary Hypertension

HEREDITY - ENVIRONMENT

	Age
PREHYPERTENSION	0-30
EARLY HYPERTENSION	20-40
ESTABLISHED HYPERTENSION	30-50

UNCOMPLICATED

COMPLICATED

Accelerated Malignant Course

CARDIAC
Hypertrophy
Failure
Infarction

LARGE VESSEL
Aneurysm
Dissection

CEREBRAL
Ischemia
Thrombosis
Hemorrhage

RENAL
Nephrosclerosis
Failure

A simplified scheme of the natural history of untreated primary hypertension

FIGURE 4.2

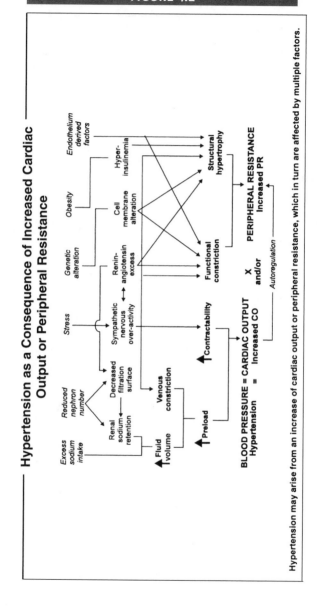

Hypertension as a Consequence of Increased Cardiac Output or Peripheral Resistance

Hypertension may arise from an increase of cardiac output or peripheral resistance, which in turn are affected by multiple factors.

TABLE 4.1

Overall Guide to Work-up for Identifiable Causes of Hypertension

Diagnosis	Diagnostic Procedure	
	Initial	Additional
Chronic renal disease	Urinalysis, serum creatinine, renal sonography	Isotopic renogram, renal biopsy
Renovascular disease	Captopril-enhanced isotopic renogram, duplex sonography	MR or CT angiogram, aortogram
Coarctation	Blood pressure in legs	Echocardiogram, aortogram
Primary aldosteronism	Plasma and urinary potassium, plasma renin and aldosterone (ratio)	Plasma or urinary aldosterone after saline load, adrenal CT and scintiscans
Cushing's syndrome	Morning plasma cortisol after 1 mg dexamethasone at bedtime	Urinary cortisol after variable doses of dexamethasone, adrenal CT and scintiscans
Pheochromocytoma	Plasma metanephrine Spot urine for metanephrine	Urinary catechols, plasma catechols (basal and after 0.3 mg clonidine), adrenal CT and scintiscans

References

Barker DJP, Shiell AW, Barker ME, Law CM: Growth in utero and blood pressure levels in the next generation. *J Hypertens* 2000;18:843–846.

Beevers G, Lip GYH, O'Brien E: The pathophysiology of hypertension. *Br Med J* 2001;322:912–916.

Black HR, Weltin G, Jaffe CC: The limited echocardiogram: A modification of standard echocardiography for use in the routine evaluation of patients with systemic hypertension. *Am J Cardiol* 1991;67:1027–1030.

Brenner BM, Chertow GM: Congenital oligonephropathy and the etiology of adult hypertension and progressive renal injury. *Am J Kidney Dis* 1994;23:171–175.

Cardillo C, Kilcoyne CM, Waclawiw M, et al.: Role of endothelin in the increased vascular tone of patients with essential hypertension. *Hypertension* 1999;33:753–758.

Field AE, Coakley EH, Must A, et al.: Impact of overweight on the risk of developing common chronic diseases during a 10-year period. *Arch Intern Med* 2001;161:1582–1586.

Isomaa B, Almgren P, Tuomi T, et al.: Cardiovascular morbidity and mortality associated with the metabolic syndrome. *Diabetes Care* 2001;24:683–689.

Kaplan NM: Anxiety-induced hyperventilation. *Arch Intern Med* 1997;157:945–948.

Park JB, Schiffrin EL: Small artery remodeling is the most prevalent (earliest?) form of target organ damage in mild essential hypertension. *J Hypertens* 2001;19:921–930.

Weber MA. The measurement of arterial properties in hypertension. *Am J Hypertens* 2001;14:183–185.

NOTES

#5 Secondary Hypertension: Renal

Renal Parenchymal Disease
Renal Vascular Hypertension (RVH)

Frequency

Beyond obesity and alcohol abuse in men, renal parenchymal and vascular diseases are the most common causes of secondary hypertension, particularly in children, the elderly, and those with severe or resistant disease.

5.

RENAL PARENCHYMAL DISEASE

Some patients who start with primary hypertension develop progressive nephrosclerosis and end up with chronic renal failure. This course is more common among black hypertensives and those who have coexisting diabetes mellitus or poorly controlled hypertension. Proteinuria is an independent mediator of renal damage, and microalbuminuria is a risk factor for all forms of CVD.

As renal function deteriorates, hypertension becomes more prominent and is present in about 85% of those with end-stage renal disease (ESRD). In such patients, it may not be possible to dissect cause from effect, but renal function is normal in most patients with primary hypertension whose BPs were well controlled, whereas renal dysfunction (proteinuria, elevated serum creatinine, lower glomerular filtration rate [GFR]) is prominent even without significant hypertension in most with a renal cause.

Clinical Features

The BP tends to rise as renal function is lost, mainly from the inability of damaged kidneys to excrete sodium and water. In some patients, renin hypersecretion is responsible, and the absence of normal renal vasodepressor hormones may be involved.

All forms of progressive renal disease may lead to hypertension, including:

- Polycystic disease (frequently)
- Analgesic nephropathy (less frequently)
- Vasculitis (as in collagen vascular disease; this may induce acute, severe renal failure)
- Pyelonephritis (rarely, except in patients with reflux nephropathy)
- Diabetic nephropathy (which is becoming more prevalent as more people become obese and as diabetics live longer)
- Obstructive nephropathy (as with BPH)

Management

More aggressive control of hypertension to levels below 120/80 mm Hg may slow or even partially reverse the progress of renal failure. In the presence of renal insufficiency, control of hypertension depends mainly on control of fluid volume, which may require:

- Restriction of dietary sodium
- High doses of loop diuretics
- Dialysis

Potent vasodilating antihypertensive agents, in particular minoxidil, may be especially useful (see Section #32). In all forms of nephropathy, angiotensin-converting enzyme inhibitors (ACEIs) and angiotensin II-receptor blockers (ARBs) appear to provide special protection against progression of renal damage (see Section #30).

RENAL VASCULAR HYPERTENSION

Clinical Features

In most patients with RVH, one or more of the following features will usually be noted:

- Onset of hypertension before age 30 or after age 50
- Rapid progression of the degree of hypertension
- A diastolic bruit lateral to the midline, just below the ribcage
- Poor response to most antihypertensive drugs
- Rapid progression of renal insufficiency after use of an ACEI or ARB usually heralds bilateral renal hypertension or stenosis of the artery to a solitary kidney. In both settings, the renal circulation is critically dependent on high levels of angiotensin II (A-II) acting on A-II receptors. If A-II is lowered or blocked, renal perfusion will be acutely reduced.

In younger patients, particularly women, medial fibroplasia is the most common form of renal vascular disease. In older patients, atherosclerotic plaques are the most common.

Diagnosis

In some patients, RVH cannot be distinguished on clinical grounds from primary hypertension. Little is lost if the diagnosis is not made in such patients, as long as their hypertension can be well controlled and usual indices of renal function (serum creatinine) remain normal.

Those with the suggestive features listed above should be evaluated for RVH. For screening of patients with less suggestive features, noninvasive procedures are recommended, either duplex ultrasonography or the captopril challenge test.

The more suggestive the features, the more essential it is to perform the definitive diagnostic test, a renal arteriogram. Magnetic resonance angiography is being increasingly used, particularly in patients with renal insufficiency. Renal vein ratios rarely are needed to establish the diagnosis in those with bilateral stenoses.

Therapy

Medical therapy, even if successful in control of hypertension, may not stop the progress of renal atrophy so that careful observation of renal function is mandatory.

Surgical repair may be preferable, particularly in younger patients. Percutaneous angioplasty has been used increasingly in initial therapy. Although lasting relief of hypertension has been obtained in fewer than one-third of patients, the results are likely improved by use of renal artery stents.

References

Chábová V, Schirger A, Stanson AW, et al.: Outcomes of atherosclerotic renal artery stenosis managed without revascularization. *Mayo Clin Proc* 2000;75:437–444.

La Batide-Alanore A, Azizi M, Froissart M, et al.: Split renal function outcome after renal angioplasty in patients with unilateral renal artery stenosis. *J Am Soc Nephrol* 2001;12: 1235–1241.

Radermacher J, Chavan A, Bleck J, et al.: Use of Doppler ultrasonography to predict the outcome of therapy for renal-artery stenosis. *N Engl J Med* 2001;344:410–417.

Rahman M, Fu P, Ashwini R, et al.: Interdialytic weight gain, compliance with dialysis regimen, and age are independent predictors of blood pressure in hemodialysis patients. *Am J Kidney Dis* 2000;35:257–265.

Ruggenenti P, Schieppati A, Remuzzi G: Progression, remission, regression of chronic renal diseases. Lancet 2001; 357:1601–1608.

Safian RD, Textor SC: Renal-artery stenosis. *N Engl J Med* 2001;344:431–442.

Tuttle KR: Ischemic nephropathy. *Curr Opin Nephrol Hypertens* 2001;10:167–173.

van Jaarsveld BC, Deinum J: Evaluation and treatment of renal artery stenosis: Impact on blood pressure and renal function. *Curr Opin Nephrol Hypertens* 2001;10:399–404.

Walls J: Relationship between proteinuria and progressive renal disease. *Am J Kidney Dis* 2001;37(Suppl 2):S13–S16.

Watson PS, Hadjipetrou P, Cox SV, et al.: Effect of renal artery stenting on renal function and size in patients with atherosclerotic renovascular disease. *Circulation* 2000;102:1671–1677.

NOTES

#6 Secondary Hypertension: Adrenal

Pheochromocytoma
Cushing's Syndrome
Primary Aldosteronism

As many as two percent of abdominal computerized tomography (CT) scans will reveal an incidental adrenal mass, usually a nonfunctioning, benign lesion. The diagnostic studies listed in Table 4.1 and additional imaging studies may be needed to rule out a functional adenoma or cancer.

6.

Types of Adrenal Hypertension

Hypertension accompanies hyperfunction of the adrenal medulla (pheochromocytoma) or cortex (Cushing's syndrome with excess cortisol or primary aldosteronism). In total, these syndromes comprise less than one percent of hypertension among adults, although recent studies suggest a much higher prevalence of primary aldosteronism. In children, hypersecretion of mineralocorticoids can be the consequence of congenital adrenal enzyme deficiencies (congenital adrenal hyperplasia). Another two rare but fascinating mechanisms for mineralocorticoid hypertension have been elucidated.

PHEOCHROMOCYTOMA

Clinical Features

The types and approximate frequency of occurrence of tumors are:
- Unilateral, benign—80 percent
- Malignant—10 percent
- Bilateral, benign—10 percent

Bilateral benign tumors are often part of the multiple endocrine neoplasia (MEN-2) syndrome accompanied by medullary cancer of the thyroid. In both MEN-2 and von Hippel-Landau familial syndromes, the clinical manifestations of pheochromocytomas may be absent.

The hypertension may be episodic or sustained, but intermittent spells are almost always noted that include:

- Headache
- Tachycardia
- Sweating
- Tremor

The excess catecholamines usually induce a hypermetabolic state with:

- Weight loss
- Hyperglycemia
- Intense peripheral vasoconstriction with paleness

Diagnosis

Patients with widely fluctuating BPs and repeated spells should have a plasma or spot urine metanephrine assay. If the metanephrine is only slightly elevated, documentation may be obtained by measurement of plasma catecholamines, first with the patient in a basal state and then three hours after 0.3 mg of clonidine, which will suppress catecholamine secretion from normal adrenals but not from pheochromocytomas. Falsely high levels with all these tests may occur if patients are receiving labetalol.

An abdominal CT scan will usually demonstrate the tumor. Metaiodobenzylguanidine isotopic scans and positron emission tomography with various isotopes may be used for those not identified by CT.

Therapy

Surgery should be performed after the manifestations of catecholamine excess are reversed by alpha-receptor blockade, preferably with dibenzyline and, if tachycardia is prominent, the addition of a beta-blocker. Laparoscopic surgery is being more widely used when tumors are accurately localized.

CUSHING'S SYNDROME

Clinical Features

Hypertension is present in approximately 85 percent of patients with Cushing's syndrome whether it is caused by:

- Bilateral adrenal hyperplasia from adrenocorticotropic hormone (ACTH) hypersecretion from the pituitary or an ectopic tumor
- A benign adrenal tumor
- An adrenal carcinoma

Cortisol excess is usually manifested by:
- Redistribution of body fat (truncal obesity)
- Decrease in protein synthesis (thin skin with striae and ecchymoses, osteoporosis)
- Increase in glucose synthesis (hyperglycemia)

Diagnosis

Measurement of plasma cortisol obtained the morning after a 1 mg dose of dexamethasone at bedtime is an excellent screening test, with almost all non-Cushing's patients suppressing below 7 μg/dl. Documentation of the type of Cushing's can be made by more prolonged administration of varying doses of dexamethasone, measuring 24-hour urine cortisol levels. Plasma ACTH levels and CT scans will provide additional confirmation of the type of Cushing's and may supplant the prolonged dexamethasone suppression tests. If these studies are ambiguous, bilateral inferior petrossal sinus sampling for ACTH levels may be needed.

Therapy

The cause of the cortisol excess, either from the pituitary in those with bilateral hyperplasia or from an adrenal tumor, should be surgically removed. Various inhibitors of cortisol synthesis are available to prepare for surgery or to provide at least partial control for those in whom surgery is not feasible.

PRIMARY ALDOSTERONISM

In multiple series of presumably unselected hypertensives tested by a plasma aldosterone to renin ratio (ARR), the prevalence of primary aldosteronism has been reported to be as high as 20 percent. More than half are normokalemic. Since most of these patients turn out to have bilateral adrenal hyperplasia, there seems little need for such screening in most patients.

Clinical Features

Mineralocorticoid excess may arise from a solitary benign adenoma or bilateral hyperplasia. In general, secretion is greater from an adenoma, so the manifestations are more severe:

- Plasma potassium is lower
- Plasma renin activity (PRA) is lower
- Plasma and urine aldosterone is higher

The syndrome should be considered in hypertensives with hypokalemia that is not provoked by diuretics, gastrointestinal (GI) losses, etc. Almost all patients will have hypertension, which is often severe in degree, and hypokalemia, which may be intermittent (Figure 6.1).

Diagnosis

In hypokalemic hypertensives, the finding of urinary potassium wastage of more then 30 mmol per day in the face of low plasma K^+ is a useful initial screening test if the urine is collected without sodium restriction or potassium supplementation. If a blood sample contains high aldosterone (<20 ng/dl) and low renin activity (<1 ng/ml/hr), providing an ARR > 50, primary aldosteronism is likely. Autonomous hypersecretion of aldosterone may be demonstrated by failure to suppress plasma aldosterone below 6 ng/dl after 2 liters of intravenous (IV) normal saline over four hours or urinary aldosterone to <14 μg/d after 3 days of oral salt loading. CT scans will usually demonstrate the adrenal pathology, but a number of special procedures may be needed for additional confirmation if a solitary tumor is not seen. In particular, adrenal vein sampling is being used for those with ambiguous scans.

Therapy

Adenomas should be surgically removed. Bilateral hyperplasia should be controlled with the aldosterone antagonist spironolactone. If that is poorly tolerated, amiloride or triamterene will usually correct the hypokalemia. A thiazide diuretic may also be needed.

Apparent Mineralocorticoid Excess

Apparent mineralocorticoid excess (i.e., hypertension and/or hypokalemia but low levels of aldosterone) can be induced by inhibition of the 11-β-hydroxysteroid dehydrogenase (11-β-OHSD) enzyme that normally converts cortisol (which binds to the renal mineralocorticoid receptor) to cortisone (which does not bind). The persistent high level of cortisol in the kidney acts as a potent mineralocorticoid. The glycyrrhizic acid present in licorice (now frequently added to chewing tobacco) will inhibit the enzyme and induce the syndrome. A few cases of idiopathic 11-β-OHSD deficiency have been identified. Ulick et al. have also identified an abnormality in the peripheral metabolism of cortisol, which is the more common mechanism for this syndrome.

Glucocorticoid-Suppressible Aldosteronism

Multiple families have been recognized with members having mineralocorticoid excess that is suppressible by dexamethasone. Lifton et al. have identified a genetic crossover of the genes for the aldosterone synthetase enzyme (normally only in the outer zona glomerulosa and not influenced by ACTH) and the 11-hydroxylase enzyme (normally in the middle zona fasciculata and influenced by ACTH). The excess aldosterone synthetase results in synthesis of high levels of mineralocorticoids from the ACTH-responsive zona fasciculata. Partial defects could be involved in more patients with "low-renin" hypertension.

FIGURE 6.1

The Pathophysiology of
Primary Aldosteronism

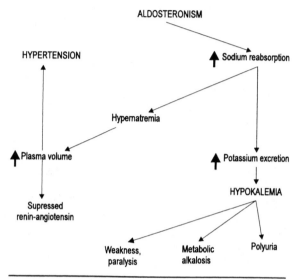

The pathophysiology of primary aldosteronism (from Kaplan N.M.: *Clinical Hypertension*, 8th ed., Philadelphia: Lippincott Williams & Wilkins.

References

Adrenal Incidentalomas

Luton JP, Martinez M, Bertherat J: Outcome in patients with adrenal incidentaloma selected for surgery: An analysis of 88 cases investigated in a single clinical center. *Eur J Endocrinol* 2000;143:111–117.

Pheochromocytoma

Pacak K, Eisenhofer G, Carrasquillo JA, et al.: 6-[^{18}F]Fluorodopamine positron emission tomographic (PET) scanning for diagnostic localization of pheochromocytoma. *Hypertension* 2001;38:6–8.

Pacak K, Linehan WM, Eisenhofer G, et al.: Recent advances in genetics, diagnosis, localization, and treatment of pheochromocytoma. *Ann Intern Med* 2001;134:315–329.

Prys-Roberts C: Phaeochromocytoma-Recent progress in its management. *Br J Anaesth* 2000;85:44–57.

Roden M, Raffesberg W, Raber W, et al.: Quantification of unconjugated metanephrines in human plasma without interference by acetaminophen. *Clin Chem* 2001;47:1061–1067.

Cushing's Syndrome

Boscaro M, Barzon L, Fallo F, Sonino N: Cushing's syndrome. *Lancet* 2001;357:783–791.

Montwill J, Igoe D, McKenna TJ: The overnight dexamethasone test is the procedure of choice in screening for Cushing's syndrome. *Steroids* 1994;59:296–298.

Primary Aldosteronism

Kaplan NM: Cautions over the current epidemic of primary aldosteronism. *Lancet* 2001;357:953–954.

Lifton RP, Dluhy RG, Powers M, et al.: A chimaeric 11β-hydroxylase/aldosterone synthase gene causes glucocorticoid-remediable aldosteronism and human hypertension. *Nature* 1992;355:262–265.

Lim PO, Young WF, MacDonald TM: A review of the medical treatment of primary aldosteronism. *J Hypertens* 2001;19: 353–361.

Rich GM, Ulick S, Cook S, et al.: Glucocorticoid-remediable aldosteronism in a large kindred: Clinical spectrum and diagnosis using a characteristic biochemical phenotype. *Ann Intern Med* 1992;116:813–820.

Rossi GP, Sacchetto A, Chiesura-Corona M, et al.: Identification of the etiology of primary aldosteronism with adrenal vein sampling in patients with equivocal computed tomography and magnetic resonance findings: Results in 104 consecutive cases. *J Clin Endocrinol Metab* 2001;86:1083–1090.

Stewart PM, Corrie JET, Shackleton CHL, Edwards CRW: Syndrome of apparent mineralocorticoid excess: A defect in the cortisol-cortisone shuttle. *J Clin Invest* 1988;82:340–349.

Stewart PM: Dexamethasone-suppressible hypertension. *Lancet* 2000;356:697–699.

Stowasser M: Primary aldosteronism: Rare bird or common cause of secondary hypertension? *Curr Hypertens Rep* 2001;3:230–239.

Ulick S, Tedde R, Wang JZ: Defective ring A reduction of cortisol as a major metabolic error in the syndrome of apparent mineralocorticoid excess. *J Clin Endocrinol Metab* 1992;74: 593–599.

Weinberger MH, Fineberg NS: The diagnosis of primary aldosteronism and separation of two major subtypes. *Arch Intern Med* 1993;153:2125–2129.

White PC: Disorders of aldosterone biosynthesis and action. *N Engl J Med* 1994;331:250–258.

NOTES

#7 Secondary Hypertension: Estrogen and Pregnancy

Estrogen-Induced Hypertension
Pregnancy Hypertension

As many as five percent of women who take estrogen-containing OCs and a somewhat smaller percentage of pregnant women will develop reversible hypertension. The first situation contributes to vascular complications of OCs; the second is a major cause of fetal mortality.

Postmenopausal estrogen replacement therapy does not cause hypertension and can be safely given to hypertensive women.

7.

ESTROGEN-INDUCED HYPERTENSION

Clinical Features

The BP rises a few mm Hg in most women who take estrogen-containing OCs. About five percent of patients will have BPs that rise beyond 140/90 mm Hg within five years. If OCs are stopped, hypertension will recede in about two-thirds of this five percent. The remaining one-third either will have underlying primary hypertension or will have suffered vascular damage that sustains the OC-induced rise in BP.

The hypertension is usually mild but rarely induces severe renal vascular damage. The mechanism for the hypertension is uncertain but may involve estrogen-induced increases in renin substrate that somehow cause increased A-II levels. Hypertension is less common with the use of OCs with low doses of estrogen.

Management

Women older than age 35 should not use OCs, particularly if they smoke cigarettes. When used for temporary birth control in younger women, OCs are quite safe.

The BP should be monitored every three to six months. If hypertension develops, another form of contraceptive should be substituted.

PREGNANCY HYPERTENSION

Clinical Features

During pregnancy, hypertension may be noted early, when it usually represents primary hypertension, or late, when it usually represents the self-limited process, gestational or pregnancy-induced hypertension (PIH). The latter, if accompanied by proteinuria and edema, is called pre-eclampsia; if encephalopathy and convulsions ensue, the process is called eclampsia.

In response to vasodilation, the BP normally falls during the first and second trimesters, with levels of 100/60 mm Hg commonly noted. Women who have unrecognized hypertension before pregnancy may lower their high levels enough to be no longer hypertensive. When their levels rise during the later months, they may be thought to have PIH, the self-limited disease that arises during the last trimester and disappears soon after delivery. Edema and proteinuria usually occur with PIH.

Most self-limited PIH occurs in the last few weeks of pregnancy. The majority of women with hypertension appearing before week 36 have underlying (previous) essential hypertension or renal disease.

The diagnosis of PIH has been based on a rise of more than 30/15 mm Hg or to a level above 140/90 mm Hg in the last half of pregnancy. To reduce the number of misdiagnoses of chronic hypertension as PIH, the DBP should have been measured earlier as below 90 mm Hg but to have risen at least 25 mm Hg to above 90 mm Hg.

Mechanisms

PIH is most likely to appear among:
- Young primigravidae
- Those with underlying vascular disease (e.g., diabetes, primary hypertension)
- Those with large placental masses (multiple births, moles)

These associations have suggested that the process is induced by reduced uteroplacental blood flow likely secondary to deficient trophoblastic migration, which could reflect either poor placentation or a maternal predisposition to arterial damage, referred to as acute atherosis of the placental spiral arteries. As a result, trophoblastic debris enters the maternal circulation, setting off an inflammatory response that produces diffuse endothelial cell dysfunction with decreased production of nitric oxide.

The maternal vasoconstriction may reflect other mechanisms, including reduced levels of vasodilatory prostaglandins, perhaps associated with an excess of vasoconstricting thromboxanes.

The role of prostaglandin imbalance, arising perhaps from disordered placental steroid synthesis, has been supported by reports of a reduced incidence among women considered to be at risk for PIH who were given 60 mg of aspirin per day.

Large-scale preventive trials with low doses of aspirin support this only for those at high risk.

Management of PIH

Women diagnosed as having PIH should restrict activities and be carefully monitored, occasionally in high-risk pregnancy units. Antihypertensives are given only if DBPs remain above 100 mm Hg, and diuretics are used only if congestive heart failure supervenes.

Women with chronic hypertension have been successfully managed with diuretics, methyldopa, and, more recently, beta-blockers and calcium blockers. However, small fetal size has been reported after beta-blocker use.

If eclampsia threatens, parenteral magnesium is used as an anticonvulsant and hydralazine as an antihypertensive. The overall aim of management is to allow the fetus to reach adequate maturity while protecting the mother from vascular damage.

Prevention

Avoidance of known risk factors should prevent pre-eclampsia. These include:
- Avoiding teenage pregnancy
- Reducing obesity and insulin resistance
- Providing good prenatal nutrition, including adequate calcium intake
- Avoiding multiple births during assisted pregnancies

Management of Chronic Hypertension

With the absolute contraindication of ACEIs and ARBs, most antihypertensive drugs being taken before pregnancy may be continued, including diuretics. However, the only drugs approved for use during pregnancy are methyl-dopa and hydralazine. The evidence for the value of any therapy of mild-to-moderate hypertension during pregnancy is sparse and inconclusive. Hopefully, large controlled trials will be performed.

References

Dekker G, Sibai B: Primary, secondary, and tertiary prevention of pre-eclampsia. *Lancet* 2001;357:209–215.

Duley L, Henderson-Smart D, Knight M, King J: Antiplatelet drugs for prevention of preeclampsia and its consequences. *Br Med J* 2001;322:329–333.

Ferrer RL, Sibai BM, Mulrow CD, et al.: Management of mild chronic hypertension during pregnancy: A review. *Obstet Gynecol* 2000;96:849–860.

Higgins JR, de Sweit M: Blood-pressure measurement and classification of pregnancy. *Lancet* 2001;357:131–135.

Lip GYH, Beevers M, Churchill D, Beevers DG: Hormone replacement therapy and blood pressure in hypertensive women. *J Hum Hypertens* 1994;8:491–494.

Manson JE, Martin KA: Postmenopausal hormone-replacement therapy. *N Engl J Med* 2001;345:34–40.

National HBPEP Working Group. Report of the National High Blood Pressure Education Program Working Group on High Blood Pressure in Pregnancy. *Am J Obstet Gynecol* 2000;183:S1–S22.

Paterson-Brown S, Robson SC, Redfern N, et al.: Hydralazine boluses for the treatment of severe hypertension in pre-eclampsia. *Br J Obstet Gynaecol* 1994;101:409–413.

Redman CWG, Sargent IL: Placental debris, oxidative stress and pre-eclampsia. *Placenta* 2000;21:597–602.

Umeda M, Ichikawa S, Kanda T, et al.: Hormone replacement therapy increases plasma level of angiotensin II in post-menopausal hypertensive women. *Am J Hypertens* 2001; 14:206–211.

Woods JW: Oral contraceptives and hypertension. *Hypertension* 1988;11(Suppl 2):II11–II15.

#8 Secondary Hypertension: Other Causes

Hormonal
Stress/Surgery
Neurogenic
Drugs

The large number of relatively rare forms of secondary hypertension infrequently pose either diagnostic or therapeutic difficulty. The following covers only the more common or potentially serious forms.

HORMONAL

8.

Hyperparathyroidism
Hypercalcemia from any cause may increase peripheral resistance and raise the BP. Most patients with hyperparathyroidism are hypertensive, although the BP becomes normal only in a minority after cure of the hyperparathyroidism.

Hypothyroidism
The DBP may be increased from peripheral vasoconstriction, but the systolic level is usually not increased, since cardiac output is reduced. Streeten et al. found a surprisingly high 3.6 percent of hypertensives to be hypothyroid, but Bergus et al. found no association between BP and thyroid-stimulating hormone (TSH) levels.

Hyperthyroidism
The high cardiac output tends to raise systolic levels, but the diastolic is usually reduced,

presumably because of peripheral vasodilation in response to increased metabolic demands.

Acromegaly

Most patients are hypertensive, likely as a result of fluid volume excess.

Coarctation of the Aorta

This congenital defect should be looked for in all infants and children with elevated arm BP. If lower-leg BP and a systolic heart murmur are noted, echocardiography should be performed.

STRESS/SURGERY

Acute Stress and Anxiety

Marked activation of the sympathetic nervous system may induce considerable hypertension. Patients with severe chest pain from myocardial ischemia or abdominal pain from acute pancreatitis usually have significant hypertension that may rapidly recede as the pain is relieved. Caution should be taken in using potent parenteral antihypertensive agents in such patients unless their high pressures remain a threat after relief of their acute symptoms.

Transient elevations in pressure may accompany anxiety-induced acute hyperventilation. The author finds hyperventilation to be a common cause of symptoms (dizziness, paresthesias, headache) in newly diagnosed or poorly controlled hypertensives.

Postoperative

BP may rise during and after surgery in response to various stimuli, including:

- Hypoxia
- Pain
- Volume excess

A particularly high frequency of hypertension follows coronary bypass surgery, likely as a result of marked sympathetic nervous stimulation. Surgery on the carotid arteries may also be followed by significant hypertension.

Various parenteral antihypertensive agents have been used to treat perioperative hypertension. Nitroprusside is most potent but cumbersome to use; labetalol, nicardipine, or esmolol may be effective alternatives.

Burns
Many patients with third-degree burns over more than 20 percent of body surfaces will develop hypertension that may require appropriate therapy.

Hypoglycemia
The catecholamine response to insulin-induced hypoglycemia may provoke severe hypertension, particularly in patients receiving beta-blockers.

NEUROGENIC

Sleep Apnea
A significant percentage of hypertensive patients have sleep apnea, particularly if they are overweight. In most, the apnea is obstructive rather than central and therefore has been assumed to be the cause of the hypertension rather than a consequence of central nervous

system (CNS) damage. Relief of airway obstruction or use of nasal CPAP has been shown to result in lowering of BP.

Increased Intracranial Pressure
Significant hypertension can be caused by:
- Brain tumors
- Acute strokes
- Head trauma

It presumably results from irritation of vasomotor centers or disruptions of sympathetic nervous control.

Compression of Ventrolateral Medulla
Claims have been made for relief of hypertension by decompression of arteries compressing the ventrolateral medulla, but the overall evidence denies any association.

DRUGS

Cyclosporine and Tacrolimus
As many as half of patients given cyclosporine and tacrolimus (immunosuppressive drugs) will develop hypertension, even in the absence of renal damage.

Erythropoietin
Partly as a consequence of rapidly increased red cell mass and blood volume, hypertension may develop.

Sympathomimetics
Street drugs (amphetamines, cocaine) and over-the-counter drugs (phenylpropanolamine,

pseudoephedrine) may induce considerable hypertension.

Nonsteroidal Anti-Inflammatory Agents (NSAIDs)

Presumably by decreasing vasodilatory prostaglandins, NSAIDs may interefere with the efficacy of various antihypertensive drugs.

References

Bergus GR, Mold JW, Barton ED, Randall CS: The lack of association between hypertension and hypothyroidism in a primary care setting. *J Hum Hypertens* 1999;13:231–235.

Daniels SR: Repair of coarctation of the aorta and hypertension: Does age matter? *Lancet* 2001;358:89.

FitzGerald GA, Patrono C: The coxibs, selective inhibitors of cyclooxygenase-2. *N Engl J Med* 2001;345:433–442.

Hia KM, Young TB, Bidwell T, et al.: Sleep apnea and hypertension: A population-based study. *Ann Intern Med* 1994; 120:382–388.

Kaplan NM: Anxiety-induced hyperventilation. *Arch Intern Med* 1997;157:945–948.

Lange RA, Hillis LD: Cardiovascular complications of cocaine use. *N Engl J Med* 2001;345:351–358.

Lester SJ, Baggott M, Welm S, et al.: Cardiovascular effects of 3,4-methylenedioxymethamphetamine. *Ann Intern Med* 2000; 133:969–973.

Parker KP, Mitch WE, Stivelman JC, et al.: Safety and efficacy of low-dose subcutaneous erythropoietin in hemodialysis patients. *J Am Soc Nephrol* 1997;8:288–293.

Streeten DHP, Anderson GH Jr., Howland T, et al.: Effects of thyroid function on blood pressure: Recognition of hypothyroid hypertension. *Hypertension* 1988;11:78–83.

Thuerl C, Rump LC, Otto M, et al.: Neurovascular contact of the brain stem in hypertensive and normotensive subjects: MR findings and clinical significance. *Am J Neuroradiol* 2001;22: 476–480.

Wright JT Jr., Redline S, Taylor AL, et al.: Relationship between 24-h blood pressure and sleep disordered breathing in a normotensive community sample. *Am J Hypertens* 2001; 14:743–448.

#9 Lifestyle Modifications: Dietary

Weight Reduction
Sodium Reduction
Other Dietary Changes

Increasing evidence suggests that hypertension may be delayed and perhaps prevented by early and continued modification of lifestyle, including:
- Avoidance of obesity
- Moderation of sodium and alcohol
- Regular exercise

Once hypertension is present, therapy should always include a variety of nondrug therapies, better referred to as lifestyle modifications. Those involving the diet will be included in this section; others are covered in Section #10. A diet rich in fruits and vegetables and low-fat dairy foods, the DASH (Dietary Approaches to Stop Hypertension) diet, substantially lowered BPs in a short-term clinical trial (Sachs et al., 2001). In the Treatment of Mild Hypertension Study (TOMHS), modest degrees of weight reduction, sodium and alcohol restriction, and increased exercise provided a 8.6/8.6 mm Hg fall in BP over a 48-month follow-up.

WEIGHT REDUCTION

Almost half of all hypertensive people are overweight. As weight is gained, the BP usually rises; as weight is lost, the BP usually falls. Sleep apnea may be involved in a larger segment of the obese hypertensive population than now recognized, having been reported in 30 percent or more of even slightly obese hypertensives. In some, the hypertension may recede when sleep apnea is overcome.

Hyperinsulinemia is present in obese people, particularly in those whose obesity is predominantly in the abdomen and upper body. High levels of insulin may raise the BP by multiple mechanisms.

Calories should be restricted in a manner appropriate to the individual patient. For most, a 1,200 calorie low-fat diet will provide gradual weight loss without discomfort. For some, more restrictive diets may be needed. Appetite suppressants that do not cause systemic pressor effects may be helpful.

SODIUM REDUCTION

Reduction of dietary sodium to 2.4 g per day (100 mmol or 6 g of sodium chloride [NaCl]) will lower BP by 5 to 10 mm Hg in a significant number of sodium-sensitive hypertensives, including the majority of elderly and black patients. This degree of reduction can be attained by avoiding highly salted foods (e.g., pickles, processed meats, canned tomato juice) and adding no salt at the table or during cooking. Potassium chloride (KCl), either alone or with magnesium and lysine (Cardia), may be used as a salt substitute, with caution in those with renal insufficiency.

An awareness is required of the hidden sodium present in most processed foods, such as canned vegetables and many breakfast cereals (Table 9.1). Fresh or unprocessed frozen foods should be used whenever possible.

Although not all patients will respond to such moderate sodium restriction, no harm should occur from the return to the natural lower-sodium diet consumed by humans throughout history until the recent past. The reduction in sodium may reduce potassium loss if diuretics are given, and the lower-sodium fresh foods will likely have higher amounts of potassium than are present in processed forms of these foods. Moreover, a high-sodium intake is correlated with left ventricular hypertrophy (LVH) independent of BP.

More rigid sodium restriction may be needed for patients with renal failure or severe heart failure. If needed, low-sodium preparations of a number of processed foods are available (Table 9.1).

OTHER DIETARY CHANGES

Potassium Supplementation

Correction of hypokalemia may lower BP. Although supplemental KCl has been shown to lower BP in some normokalemic hypertensives, there should be little need to give such supplements if natural, high-potassium foods are substituted for the processed, high-sodium foods in the diet. Supplements of KCl may be required to replenish potassium deficiency, since dietary sources of potassium may be largely accompanied by nonreabsorbable anions, which reduce retention of potassium.

Calcium Supplementation

In a few patients, 1 to 2 g of supplemental calcium per day has been found to lower BP, but the effect is too small to support the use of such supplements for preventing or treating hypertension.

Moreover, calcium supplements increase the risk of renal stones.

Magnesium Supplementation

Magnesium supplements have not usually been noted to lower BP. However, patients who are deficient in both magnesium and potassium may not be able to replete potassium stores unless magnesium is also provided.

Other Dietary Changes

A few well-controlled studies have shown that the intake of either a lower saturated, higher unsaturated fat diet or supplements of omega-3-fatty acids will reduce BP. A fall in BP has been noted with a high-fiber diet, and higher dietary protein intake appears to be associated with lower BP.

Moderation of Alcohol

Besides adding calories, alcohol consumption may raise BP. In multiple population surveys, daily consumption of more than one ounce of alcohol per day is associated with higher BP, and more than two ounces per day is often associated with overt hypertension (see Figure 9.1). One-half to one ounce of alcohol per day will likely not raise BP but will provide protection against coronary heart disease (CHD) and mortality. One ounce of alcohol is contained in:

- Two 12 oz. beers OR
- Two 4 oz. glasses of wine OR
- Two 1.5 oz. portions of whiskey

Cardioprotection has been demonstrated in many epidemiological surveys wherein those who drink up to one ounce of alcohol per day have less CHD than those who do not drink alcohol. Women need only drink one-half an ounce of alcohol per day for cardioprotection.

Caffeine

A transient rise in BP follows consumption of the caffeine in a cup of coffee, but most surveys show no increase in CHD with increasing caffeine consumption.

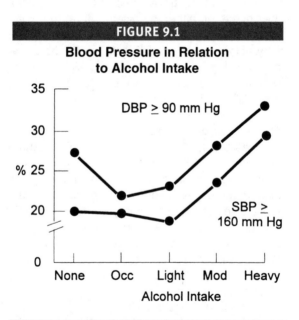

FIGURE 9.1

Blood Pressure in Relation to Alcohol Intake

Age-adjusted prevalence rates (%) of measured systolic and di-astolic hypertension by levels of alcohol intake in 7,735 English men. The levels of alcohol intake are in drinks: occasional, light (1 to 2 daily), moderate (3 to 6 daily), and heavy (more than 6 daily). (From Shaper et al.: J Hum Hypertens 1988;2:71.)

TABLE 9.1

The Sodium Content
(in milligrams) of Common Foods
(1,000 mg sodium = 44 mmol sodium)

Food	Low Na+	High Na+
Sara Lee Bagel (one)	Cinnamon Raisin = 230	Onion = 630
Pancake Mix (three 4")	Featherweight = 90	Pillsbury Extra Light = 730
Kellogg's Cereal (one cup)	Frosted Mini Wheats = 0	Product 19 = 290
Tomatoes (1/2 cup)	Fresh = 10	Catsup = 1,248
Lean Cuisine Frozen Dinners	Chicken a l'Orange = 430	Chicken Chow Mein = 980

(From DeBakey et al.: Brand Name Shopper's Guide, Master Media, New York, 1992)

References

General

Conlin PR: Dietary modification and changes in blood pressure. *Curr Opin Nephrol Hypertens* 2001;10:359–363.

Neaton JD, Grimm RH Jr., Prineas RJ, et al.: Treatment of mild hypertension study (TOMHS): Final results. *JAMA* 1993; 270:713–724.

Sachs FM, Svetkey LP, Vollmer WM, et al.: Effects on blood pressure of reduced dietary sodium and the dietary approaches to stop hypertension (DASH) diet. *N Engl J Med* 2001;344:3–10.

Whelton PK, He J, Appel L, et al.: Primary prevention of hypertension. *JAMA* 2002; 288: 1882–1888.

Weight Reduction

Després J-P, Lemieux I, Prud'homme D: Treatment of obesity: Need to focus on high risk abdominally obese patients. *Br Med J* 2001;322:716–720.

He J, Whelton PK, Appel LJ, et al.: Long-term effects of weight loss and dietary sodium reduction on incidence of hypertension. *Hypertension* 2000;35:544–549.

Masuo K, Mikami H, Ogihara T, Tuck ML: Weight reduction and pharmacologic treatment of obese hypertensives. *Am J Hypertens* 2001;14:530–538.

Stevens VJ, Obarzanek E, Cook NR, et al.: Long-term weight loss and changes in blood pressure: Results of the trials of hypertension prevention, phase II. *Ann Intern Med* 2001;134: 1–11.

Sodium Reduction

Antonios TFT, MacGregor GA: Salt: More adverse effects. *Lancet* 1996;348:250–251.

Appel LJ, Espeland MA, Easter L, et al.: Effects of reduced sodium intake on hypertension control in older individuals. *Arch Intern Med* 2001;161:685–693.

Cutler JA, Follmann D, Allender PS: Randomized trials of sodium reduction: An overview. *Am J Clin Nutr* 1997;65(Suppl): 643S–651S.

Geleijnse JM, Witteman JCM, Bak AAA, et al.: Reduction in blood pressure with a low-sodium, high-potassium, high-magnesium salt in older subjects with mild to moderate hypertension. *Br Med J* 1994;309:436–440.

Potassium Supplements

Coruzzi P, Brambilla L, Brambilla V, et al.: Potassium depletion and salt sensitivity in essential hypertension. *J Clin Endocrinol Metab* 2001;86:2857–2862.

Whelton PK, He J: Potassium in preventing and treating high blood pressure. *Semin Nephrol* 1999;19:494–499.

Calcium Supplements

Allender PS, Cutler JA, Follmann D, et al.: Dietary calcium and blood pressure: A meta-analysis of randomized clinical trials. *Ann Intern Med* 1996;124:825–831.

Griffith LE, Guyatt GH, Cook RJ, et al.: The influence of dietary and nondietary calcium supplementation on blood pressure. *Am J Hypertens* 1999;12:84–92.

Other Dietary Changes

Ferrara LA, Raimondi AS, d'Episcopo L, et al.: Olive oil and reduced need for antihypertensive medications. *Arch Intern Med* 2000;160:837–842.

Holm T, Andreassen AK, Aukrust P, et al.: Omega-3 fatty acids improve blood pressure control and preserve renal function in hypertensive heart transplant recipients. *Eur Heart J* 2001; 22:428–436.

Oberzanek E, Velletri PA, Cutler JA: Dietary protein and blood pressure. *JAMA* 1996;275:1598–1603.

Alcohol

Fagrell B, DeFaire U, Bondy S, et al.: The effects of light to moderate drinking on cardiovascular disease. *J Intern Med* 1999;246:331–340.

Fuchs FD, Chambless LE, Whelton PK, et al.: Alcohol consumption and the incidence of hypertension: The Atherosclerotic Risk in Communities study. *Hypertension* 2001;37: 1242–1250.

Klatsky AL: Should patients with heart disease drink alcohol? *JAMA* 2001;285:2004–2006.

Caffeine

Jee SH, Je J, Whelton PK, et al.: The effect of chronic coffee drinking on blood pressure. *Hypertension* 1999;33:647–652.

NOTES

#10 Lifestyle Modifications: Other

Cessation of Smoking
Dynamic Exercise
Relaxation Therapy
Overall Nondrug Program

Beyond dietary changes, other lifestyle modifications may help lower BP. These include dynamic exercise and one or another form of relaxation therapy. Claims have been made for other modalities as varied as use of chromium, acupuncture, and surgical relief of supposed brainstem compression, but their efficacies have not been shown in properly controlled clinical trials.

CESSASION OF SMOKING

Cessation of smoking is the most effective way to reduce cardiovascular risk, and that effect likely involves removal of the repeated rises in BP invoked by smoking.

10.

The transient but significant pressor effect of smoking has been missed because BP is routinely taken an hour or more after the last cigarette is smoked. As seen in Figure 10.1, smoking a cigarette acutely and markedly raises BP in long-term addicted smokers. The effect, noted over 15 minutes, is largely dissipated after 30 minutes. It is interesting (and likely one of the major reasons why coronary disease and stroke kill more smokers than cancer) that no tolerance to the nicotine stimulation of the sympathetic nervous system seems to occur.

The use of transdermal nicotine patches to help smokers quit does not have a significant effect on BP.

DYNAMIC EXERCISE

Hypertensives should be encouraged to perform regular dynamic (aerobic, isotonic) exercise. Such exercise is usually accompanied by a fall in BP, although some of this effect may reflect coincidental weight loss, changes in diet, etc.

The form of exercise is irrelevant as long as it is dynamic, i.e., involves active movement of muscles. During dynamic exercise, cardiac output rises but peripheral resistance falls from vasodilation in muscle vasculature. SBP rises but DBP tends to fall or remain the same. Static or isometric exercise, i.e., increased tension without movement, is associated with a reflex increase in both cardiac output and peripheral resistance, causing marked rises in both SBP and DBP while the isometric exercise is being performed. Nonetheless, combined dynamic and static exercise (circuit training) will also provide a long-term antihypertensive effect.

Some normotensive people have marked increases in SBP, beyond 200 mm Hg, during the intense exercise of a stress test. Data suggest that such people have a higher likelihood of subsequently developing permanent hypertension, but this is by no means invariable. Such patients should be advised to engage in gradually increasing dynamic exercise to modulate the marked systolic rise.

To reach the "conditioned" state of cardiac performance, 20 to 30 minutes of sustained exercise at 70 percent of maximal capacity, usually determined from the rise in pulse rate, is required three times each week. The level of exercise that accomplishes the greatest fall in BP has not been determined.

RELAXATION THERAPY

Almost all forms of relaxation therapy have been said to lower BP. These therapies include:
- Progressive muscle relaxation
- Yoga
- Biofeedback
- Transcendental meditation
- The Chinese breathing exercise Qi Gong
- Hypnosis

Most controlled studies have not shown a sustained effect beyond the duration of the relaxation procedure. Controlled studies have shown a lasting effect from the use of a device that slows and regularizes breathing. Those patients who seem to benefit and are willing to continue the practice of one or another relaxation therapy should be encouraged to do so.

OVERALL NONDRUG PROGRAM

The steps that should be followed as part of an overall nondrug program include:
- Stopping smoking
- Reducing body weight by caloric restriction, with cautions against use of over-the-counter appetite suppressants, most of which contain sympathomimetics that may raise BP

- Restricting dietary sodium to 2.4 g per day (100 mmol or 6 g of NaCl), about two-thirds the amount in the usual North American diet
- Maintaining adequate intake of potassium, calcium, and magnesium and supplementing these in those whose diets or levels are deficient
- Limiting alcohol intake to one ounce per day in men and one-half ounce per day in women (one ounce of alcohol is contained in two usual portions of beer, wine, or spirits)
- Performing 20 to 30 minutes of dynamic exercise at least three times a week
- Using whatever form of relaxation therapy is acceptable
- Controlling dyslipidemia, in particular with statin drugs

FIGURE 10.1

Blood Pressure After Smoking

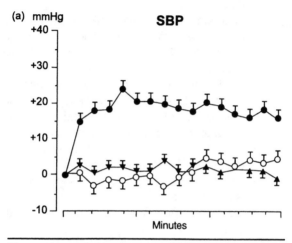

Changes in systolic blood pressure (SBP) during the first ciga-rette (●), the correspondent time of nonsmoking (○), and during sham-smoking (▲). The subjects were 10 normotensive volun-teers who were accustomed to smoking more than 20 cigarettes per day (from Groppelli et al.: J Hypertens 1992;10:495).

References

Cessation of Smoking

Groppelli A, Giorgi DMA, Omboni S, et al.: Persistent blood pressure increase induced by heavy smoking. *J Hypertens* 1992;10:495–499.

Lancaster T, Stead L, Silagy C, Sowden A: Effectiveness of interventions to help people stop smoking: Findings from the Cochrane Library. *Br Med J* 2000;321:355–358.

Raij L, DeMaster EG, Jaimes EA: Cigarette smoke-induced endothelium dysfunction: Role of superoxide anion. *J Hypertens* 2001;19:891–897.

Regalado M, Wesson DE, Yang S: Cigarette smoking is associated with augmented progression of renal insufficiency in severe essential hypertension. *Am J Kidney Dis* 2000; 35:687–692.

Tanus-Santos JE, Toledo JCY, Cittadino M, et al. Cardiovascular effects of transdermal nicotine in mildly hypertensive smokers. *Am J Hypertens* 2001;14:610–614.

Dynamic Exercise

Blair SN, Kampert JB, Kohk III HW, et al.: Influences of cardiorespiratory fitness and other precursors on cardiovascular disease and all-cause mortality in men and women. *JAMA* 1996;276:205–210.

Blumenthal JA, Sherwood A, Gullette ECD, et al.: Exercise and weight loss reduce blood pressure in men and women with mild hypertension. *Arch Intern Med* 2000;160:1947–1958.

Kelley GA, Kelley KS: Progressive resistance exercise and resting blood pressure. *Hypertension* 2000;35:838–843.

Ohkubo T, Hozawa A, Nagatomi R, et al.: Effects of exercise training on home blood pressure values in older adults: A randomized controlled trial. *J Hypertens* 2001;19:1045–1052.

Taylor-Tolbert NS, Dengel DR, Brown MB, et al.: Ambulatory blood pressure after acute exercise in older men with essential hypertension. *Am J Hypertens* 2000;13:44–51.

Relaxation Therapy

Linden W, Lenz JW, Con AH: Individualized stress management for primary hypertension. *Arch Intern Med* 2001;161: 1071–1080.

Schein MH, Gavish B, Herz M, et al.: Treating hypertension with a device that slows and regularizes breathing: A randomized, double-blind controlled study. *J Hum Hypertens* 2001;15:271–278.

Shapiro D, Hui KK, Oakley ME, et al.: Reduction in drug requirements for hypertension by means of a cognitive-behavioral intervention. *Am J Hypertens* 1997;10:9–17.

Overall Program

Borghi C, Veronesi M, Prandin MG, et al. Statins and blood pressure regulation. *Curr Hypertens Rep* 2001;3:281–288.

Whelton PK, He J, Appel L, et al.: Primary prevention of hypertension. *JAMA* 2002; 288: 1882–1888.

NOTES

#11 The Decision to Use Drugs

Evidence-Based Medicine
Steps in the Decision Process
The Issue of Protection
The Issue of Side Effects
A More Rational Approach

EVIDENCE-BASED MEDICINE

In the last few years, the need to base thera-peutic decisions on firm evidence, usually from systematic review of multiple randomized clinical trials, has been widely accepted. Such evidence-based medicine has also recognized the need to identify the benefits of therapy not on relative reductions in risk but on absolute reductions. Thus, a reduction of strokes from two per 1,000 to one per 1,000 is a 50 percent decrease in relative risk but only a 0.1 percent decrease in absolute risk. A reduction from 200 strokes per 1,000 to 100 per 1,000 is also a 50 percent decrease in rel-ative risk but a 10 percent decrease in absolute risk. The issue is nicely demonstrated by the results from the six major clinical trials of treat-ment of elderly hypertensives wherein the relative reductions were similar in all trials but the absolute reductions were progressively greater the higher the degree of risk in the untreated (placebo) populations (see Figure 11.1).

STEPS IN THE DECISION PROCESS

With evidence based on the absolute effects from randomized clinical trials, it is obvious that many patients with uncomplicated Stage 1 hypertension (defined as DBP between 90 and 100 mm Hg) who comprise the largest portion of the nonelderly population with elevated BP may not need to be immediately started on antihypertensive drugs. Although immediate start of therapy has become common practice, a more conservative approach is recommended for the following reasons.

First, such patients are at little short-term risk and will not be endangered by postponement of drug therapy until the permanence of their hypertension is ascertained by two or three months of repeated measurements. (If they become normotensive, they should remain under surveillance, since they are more likely to become hypertensive in the future.)

Second, nondrug therapies may bring and keep their BPs down. This was shown in the TOMHS (Neaton et al., 1993), wherein a rather small degree of sodium restriction, weight loss, moderation of alcohol, and increased physical activity resulted in an 8.6/8.6 mm Hg fall in BP over a 48-month follow-up.

Third, and most importantly, all drug therapies have risks, costs, and side effects. Though these may be minimized, they cannot be completely avoided.

THE ISSUE OF PROTECTION

Despite their risks, drugs would be indicated for more patients if there was clear evidence that they protected against major cardiovascular morbidity and mortality in low-risk patients to the extent that is predicted from epidemiological data.

A number of large clinical trials have demonstrated full protection against stroke. But protection against coronary disease, the most frequent and serious complication associated with hypertension, was not found to be equal to that expected.

The failure to demonstrate full protection against coronary disease in the earlier trials may reflect the manner by which the pressure was lowered. In most, large doses of diuretics were the first and often the only drugs used. In three reported trials of elderly hypertensives, the use of lower doses of diuretics has been shown to provide greater protection against coronary mortality. Moreover, in the Framingham cohort, progressively greater reductions in cardiovascular mortality have been noted among hypertensives treated in the 1980s compared with previous decades.

Another reason for the failure to show protection against coronary mortality has been suggested: the inadvertent reduction of BP to below the critical level needed to maintain myocardial perfusion, mostly in patients who have pre-existing coronary artery disease (CAD). This threshold level, in most trials, has been a DBP of 85 mm Hg, which could produce a J-curve, with increases in coronary mortality when BPs are lowered below that level by therapy.

More recent trials have shown excellent protection against stroke, heart attack, and heart failure with both calcium-channel blockers (CCBs) and ACEIs compared to placebo, whereas there has been little difference when these newer agents were compared to low-dose diuretic-based therapy.

THE ISSUE OF SIDE EFFECTS

In most of the large clinical trials, from 20 to 40 percent of patients started on drug therapy stopped it, about half because of side effects. Most side effects are mild and often only transient, and quality-of-life (QOL) measures show little or no overall impairment. However, impotence is increased, particularly among those who take diuretics.

A MORE RATIONAL APPROACH

As most vividly portrayed in the Framingham Heart Study, which has been ongoing for decades, multiple risk factors have an additive effect on the likelihood of developing CHD (see Figure 11.2). In addition to hypertension, the major risk factors are an elevated plasma cholesterol concentration, a low HDL-cholesterol concentration, diabetes mellitus, cigarette smoking, and LVH by electrocardiogram. Thus, individual patients who have significant hypertension but none or few of the other risk factors are at relatively less risk than are patients with less hypertension but more of the other risk factors.

A group of New Zealand physicians were the first to take these risk factors into account by determining the overall risk status of individual patients, along with their level of BP, age, and gender. They then examined the evidence of benefits of antihypertensive therapy from the clinical trials and considered the costs of such therapy, concluding that antihypertensive therapy can be justified only if the risk for a major cardiovascular event over the next 10 years was 20 percent or greater or if the level of BP was so high as to mandate therapy regardless of overall risk status (≥170/100). This approach requires that age, gender, and a number of cardiovascular risk factors be taken into account when considering when hypertension should be treated; the risk is lowest in younger patients, women, and those with no other risk factors, target-organ damage, or clinical CVD (see Table 11.1).

Most physicians in the United States are probably unwilling to be as conservative as the New Zealand nomogram recommends. They would almost certainly begin antihypertensive therapy in most patients with an overall 10-year risk of 10 percent or greater. Nonetheless, the concept of taking all risk factors into account seems to be a more rational basis for deciding upon the need for therapy than using one level of BP for all patients. This principle constitutes the basis of the recommendations for risk stratification and treatment of hypertension proposed by the sixth JNC report (see Table 11.2).

As seen in Table 11.2, cardiovascular risk factors must be taken into account when deciding upon proper treatment in a patient with mild hypertension. Lifestyle modifications should be recommended in all patients with even occasional BPs above 140 mm Hg systolic or 90 mm Hg diastolic. Antihypertensive drugs should be instituted if, after several repeated BP measurements, the average BP is above 160 mm Hg systolic or 100 mm Hg diastolic. At least some of these measurements should be made out of the office to avoid unnecessary treatment of "white-coat" hypertension. Drug therapy should be considered for pressures below 140 mm Hg systolic or 90 mm Hg diastolic in patients with additional risk factors or target-organ damage. These high-risk patients (e.g., diabetics with protein-uria) should be started on drug therapy at even lower levels of BP, as low as 130/80.

FIGURE 11.1

Comparison of Proportionate (Relative) and Absolute Benefit from Reduction in Incidence of Stroke

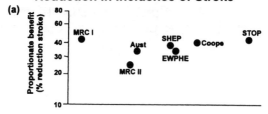

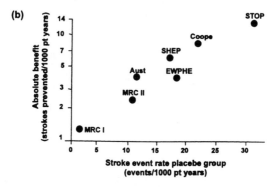

Comparison of proportionate (relative) and absolute benefit from reduction in incidence of stroke in six trials of the treatment of hypertension in the elderly and in one other with similar design but in which the absolute risk of stroke was much lower, the MRC I trial. Event rates are for fatal and nonfatal stroke combined.

Figure Abbreviations:
MRC I = Medical Research Council Trial I
MRC II = Medical Research Council Trial II
Aust = Australian Study
SHEP = Systolic Hypertension in the Elderly Program
EWPHE = European Working Party on High Blood Pressure in the Elderly Trial
Coope = Coope and Warrender
STOP = Swedish Trial in Old Patients with Hypertension

Source: Lever AF, Ramsey LE: Treatment of hypertension in the elderly. J Hypertens 1995;13:571-579.

FIGURE 11.2

Importance of multiple risk factors
for coronary disease

Estimated 10-year risk of coronary heart disease in hypothetical 55-year-old men and women according to levels of various risk factors. The risk rises gradually from below 10 percent in subjects with no risk factors to approximately 55 percent in those with six risk factors. Lipid units are in mg/dL. (Redrawn from Wilson PW, Am J Hypertens 1994;7:7S.)

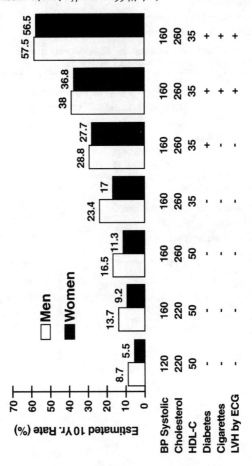

TABLE 11.1

Components for Risk Stratification in Patients with Hypertension

Major Risk Factors

Smoking

Dyslipidemia

Diabetes mellitus

Age older than 60 years

Gender (men and postmenopausal women)

Family history of cardiovascular disease (women younger than age 65 and men younger than age 55)

Target Organ Damage/Clinical Cardiovascular Disease

Heart diseases:
- Left ventricular hypertrophy
- Angina/Prior myocardial infarction
- Prior coronary revascularization
- Heart failure

Stroke or transient ischemic attack

Nephropathy

Peripheral arterial disease

Retinopathy

TABLE 11.2

Risk Stratification and Treatment*

Blood Pressure Stages (mm Hg)	Risk Group A	Risk Group B	Risk Group C
	No risk factors No TOD/CCD† (See Table 11.1)	*At least one risk factor not including diabetes mellitus No TOD/CCD† (See Table 11.1)*	*TOD/CCD† and/or diabetes mellitus with or without other risk factors (See Table 11.1)*
High to Normal (130 to 139/85 to 89 mm Hg)	Lifestyle modification	Lifestyle modification**	Drug therapy‡
Stage 1 (140 to 159/90 to 99 mm Hg)	Lifestyle modification (up to 12 months)	Lifestyle modification (up to six months)	Drug therapy
Stages 2 and 3 (≥ 160/≥ 100)	Drug therapy	Drug therapy	Drug therapy

* Lifestyle modification should be adjunctive therapy for all patients recommended for pharmacologic therapy.

** For patients with multiple risk factors, clinicians should consider drugs as initial therapy plus lifestyle modifications.

† = TOD/CCD = Target organ disease/clinical cardiovascular disease

‡ = For those with heart failure or renal insufficiency or those with diabetes mellitus

References

Alderman MH: Absolute cardiovascular risk: The basis for deciding to treat. *Am J Nephrol* 1996;16:182–189.

Blood Pressure Lowering Trialists. Effects of ACE inhibitors, calcium antagonists, and other blood-pressure-lowering drugs: Results of prospectively designed overviews of randomized trials. *Lancet* 2000;355:1955–1964.

Grimm RH, Grandits GA, Prineas RJ, et al.: Long-term effects on sexual function of five antihypertensive drugs and nutritional hygienic treatment in hypertensive men and women. Treatment of mild hypertension study (TOMHS). *Hypertension* 1997;29:8–14.

Jackson R, Barham P, Bills J, et al.: Management of raised blood pressure in New Zealand: A discussion document. *Br Med J* 1993;307:107–110.

Joint National Committee. The sixth report of the Joint National Committee on Detection, Evaluation, and Treatment of Blood Pressure (JNC-VI). *Arch Intern Med* 1997;157: 2413–2446.

Miura K, Daviglus ML, Dyer AR, et al.: Relationship of blood pressure to 25-year mortality due to coronary heart disease, cardiovascular diseases, and all causes in young adult men: The Chicago Heart Association Detection Project in Industry. *Arch Intern Med* 2001;161:1501–1508.

Mulrow CD, Pignone M: What are the elements of good treatment for hypertension? *Br Med J* 2001;322:1107–1109.

Padwal R, Straus SE, McAlister FA: Cardiovascular risk factors and their effects on the decision to treat hypertension: Evidence based review. *Br Med J* 2001;322:977–980.

Sackett DL, Rosenberg WM, Gray JAM, et al.: Evidence-based medicine: What it is and what it isn't. *Br Med J* 1996; 312:71–77.

Sytkowski PA, D'Agostino RB, Belanger AJ, Kannel WB: Secular trends in long-term sustained hypertension, long-term treatment, and cardiovascular mortality. *Circulation* 1996;93: 697–703.

NOTES

#12 Guidelines to Improve Adherence to Drug Therapy

Hypertension is adequately controlled in fewer than 25 percent of patients in the United States. More than one-third of hypertensives remain unaware of their diagnosis, and almost 20 percent who are aware are not being treated. However, almost one-third are being treated but remain uncontrolled. Thus, physician noncompliance is as much a problem as is patient noncompliance.

Patient Compliance
As many as half of patients who begin antihypertensive therapy may not be taking it one year later. Most of them simply stop the medication because of:
- Inadequate follow-up
- Lack of perceived benefit
- Side effects

Care must be taken to prescribe drugs in a way that:
- Can be easily remembered by asymptomatic people
- Will interfere as little as possible with various activities
- Will cause few side effects

12.

Therapeutic Guidelines
Guidelines that should help improve patient compliance to therapy include:
- Establishing the goal of therapy, i.e., to reduce BP below 140/90 mm Hg with minimal

or no side effects, using caution in achieving this goal in patients with known coronary disease to avoid the J-curve
- Educating patients about the disease and its treatment
- Maintaining contact with patients by:
  - Establishing visits and calls to allied health personnel
  - Making contact with patients who do not return
- Keeping care inexpensive and simple by:
  - Doing the least work-up needed to rule out secondary causes
  - Obtaining follow-up laboratory data only yearly unless indicated more often
  - Using home BP readings
  - Using nondrug, no-cost therapies
  - Using the fewest daily doses of drugs needed
  - Using combination tablets when appropriate
- Prescribing according to pharmacological principles by:
  - Adding one drug at a time
  - Starting with small doses and aiming for 5 to 10 mm Hg reductions at each step
  - Preventing volume overload with adequate diuretic and sodium reduction
  - Stopping unsuccessful therapy and trying different approaches
  - If therapy is only partially successful, adding drugs of different classes, preferably one at a time, in sufficient doses
  - Anticipating side effects
- Adjusting therapy to ameliorate side effects that do not spontaneously disappear

- Being aware of the problem and being alert to signs of patients' nonadherence and having patients bring medications to the office so that pill counts and checks on numbers of refills can be done if the BP has not responded.

The measurement of resistant hypertension is discussed in Section #28.

References

Freis ED: Improving treatment effectiveness in hypertension. *Arch Intern Med* 1999;159:2517–2521.

Haynes RB, McKibbon KA, Kanani R: Systematic review of randomized trials of interventions to assist patients to follow prescriptions for medications. *Lancet* 1996;348:383–386.

Hyman DJ, Pavlik VN: Characteristics of patients with uncontrolled hypertension in the United States. *N Engl J Med* 2001; 345:479–486.

Kaplan NM: The appropriate goals of antihypertensive therapy: Neither too much, nor too little. *Ann Intern Med* 1992;116: 686–690.

Kaplan NM: What is goal blood pressure for the treatment of hypertension? *Arch Intern Med* 2001;161:1480–1482.

Newell SA, Bowman JA, Cockburn JD: A critical review of interventions to increase compliance with medication-taking, obtaining medication refills, and appointment-keeping in the treatment of cardiovascular disease. *Prev Med* 1999;29: 535–548.

Nuesch R, Schroeder K, Dieterle T, et al.: Relation between insufficient response to antihypertensive treatment and poor compliance with treatment: A prospective case-control study. *Br Med J* 2001;323: 142–146.

#13 Diuretics: Thiazides

Clinical Information
Side Effects

CLINICAL INFORMATION

Since their introduction in the late 1950s, diuretics have been either the first or second most commonly prescribed drug for the treatment of hypertension. Even though some patients can be effectively treated without diuretics, they remain an essential element of effective therapy in most patients.

Types

Thiazides are sulfonamide derivatives that cause as much as five to eight percent of the filtered sodium load to be excreted by blocking reabsorption in the early distal tubule at the cortical diluting segment. They differ in durations of action, which, in turn, can alter the degree of metabolic side effects. Because their modes of action and potencies are similar, they share the same types of side effects (see Table 13.1).

Chemical additions to the thiazide structure provide chlorthalidone (Hygroton), with more prolonged action, and indapamide (Lozol), with some additional effects on peripheral resistance and a lesser propensity to raise serum cholesterol.

Metolozone (Mykrox, Zaroxolyn) also has effects within the proximal tubule, so it is a more potent diuretic that will work even in the presence of significant renal insufficiency.

13.

Mode of Action

To lower BP, diuretics must initially induce a natriuresis that shrinks blood volume. This activates various mechanisms responsible for maintenance of fluid volume, particularly the renin-angiotensin-aldosterone system, which, in turn, limits the degree of volume depletion.

At the same time, continued diuretic use leads to a fall in peripheral vascular resistance, which is the major reason for the continued antihypertensive effect.

Most patients achieve a 10 mm Hg fall in BP with daily diuretic therapy. Those with more "volume-dependent" hypertension, as demonstrable by lower levels of PRA, tend to respond particularly well. These patients include many black and elderly hypertensives.

Doses

Thiazides have a fairly flat dose-response curve, so that most of the antihypertensive effect is achieved with low doses (see Table 13.2). Even though as much as 200 mg of hydrochlorothiazide (HCT) per day has been used in the past, as little as 12.5 mg given once a day (the equivalent to 1.25 mg of bendrofluazide [see Table 13.2]) will provide most of the BP-lowering effect and less of the metabolic side effects of larger doses. When added to other drugs, as little as 6.25 mg may be effective (Frishman et al., 1994).

Despite having only a 12- to 18-hour duration of action, a single morning dose of HCT will provide a sustained antihypertensive effect while reducing potassium wastage during the nighttime.

Causes for Resistance

If an inadequate response is observed with 12.5 mg of HCT, the dose can be increased to 50 mg or more, although little additional effect usually is seen above 50 mg per day. The poor response may reflect either an overwhelming load of dietary sodium or an impaired renal capacity to excrete the sodium. Patients with serum creatinine above 2.0 mg/dl likely will not respond to thiazides in usual doses.

Overly vigorous diuretic therapy may activate the renin-angiotensin-aldosterone mechanism excessively. Thereby, the antihypertensive effect of the diuretic may be antagonized by the vasoconstrictive effect of angiotensin, and potassium wastage may be increased by the aldosterone-mediated exchange of more potassium for sodium.

When more severely hypertensive patients are given progressively more therapy, the reduction in BP may lead to more intense reactive sodium retention, mandating the use of additional diuretics. This has been noted particularly with the use of minoxidil, even more so when it is given to patients with renal insufficiency.

SIDE EFFECTS

A number of side effects may accompany the use of diuretics. Despite the long list of potential problems, diuretics have proven to be effective and generally safe when used in the lowest dose needed and with proper surveillance of biochemical changes.

Some side effects are allergic or idiosyncratic, such as skin rash and pancreatitis. More common effects include a variety of biochemical changes, which in large part reflect an exaggeration of the expected, desired effect of the drugs (see Figure 13.1). Though their manifestations may not be clinically obvious, they pose more serious potential hazards during the extended length of time these drugs may be used.

Hypokalemia

Urine potassium wastage is usually increased with diuretic therapy, particularly with higher doses and a high dietary sodium intake. By blocking reabsorption of NaCl in the distal tubule, the diuretic causes additional tubular fluid containing sodium to be delivered to the lower portion of the nephron wherein potassium (K^+) exchange for sodium occurs. The largest amount of potassium wastage occurs initially while the diuresis is maximal, but it may continue as long as the renin-aldosterone system is activated and sodium is delivered to the distal tubule.

The degree of renal K^+ wastage and subsequent fall in serum K^+ are largely dependent on the dose of diuretic (see Table 13.2). Diuretic-induced hypokalemia rarely causes symptoms, although muscular weakness and leg cramps may be noted. However, an increase in ventricular ectopic activity has been observed with high doses, and this may be responsible for the excess rates of sudden death observed in some of the earlier clinical trials wherein diuretic-induced hypokalemia was frequently noted and often not treated.

Hypokalemia may also be responsible for diuretic-induced glucose intolerance and hypercholesterolemia.

Diuretic-induced hypokalemia can be minimized by:

- Using the smallest dose of diuretic possible
- Using moderately long-acting diuretics, such as HCT, rather than longer-acting ones
- Reducing dietary sodium intake to 2.4 g (100 mmol) per day
- Increasing dietary potassium intake
- Combining potassium sparers with diuretics (see Section #14)
- Using drugs that suppress the renin system, e.g., beta-blockers or ACEIs or ARBs

Hypercholesterolemia

With high doses of diuretic, as much as a 10 to 20 mg/dl increase in total serum and LDL-cholesterol may develop and persist unless countered by reduction of saturated fat in the diet. The atherogenic potential of diuretic-induced rises in serum cholesterol has not been proven but probably is similar to "naturally" occurring hypercholesterolemia.

Glucose Intolerance and Hyperinsulinemia

Fasting and postprandial blood sugars may rise, but overt hyperglycemia is rare, even in patients with pre-existing diabetes. A further rise in blood insulin levels has been noted, reflecting an apparent aggravation of the peripheral insulin resistance that may accompany hypertension.

Hyperuricemia

Increased tubular reabsorption of uric acid accompanies the shrinkage of fluid volume. Diuretic-induced hyperuricemia need not be treated even if plasma levels rise above 10 mg/dl, unless gout occurs. If therapy is needed, the uricosuric agent probenecid is appropriate.

Hypercalcemia

More calcium is reabsorbed in a manner similar to uric acid, usually raising serum calcium levels by less than 0.5 mg/dl. Overt hypercalcemia may occur in patients with pre-existing unrecognized hyperparathyroidism. A decrease in calcium-containing renal stones and an increase in bone calcium content accompanies the use of thiazide diuretics.

Hyponatremia

A significant fall in plasma sodium is noted rarely, usually in elderly patients who are overdiuresed.

Hypomagnesemia

Magnesium wastage may accompany potassium wastage, and hypomagnesemia occasionally develops.

FIGURE 13.1

Side Effects of Diuretics

Mechanisms by Which Chronic Diuretic Therapy May Lead to Various Complications

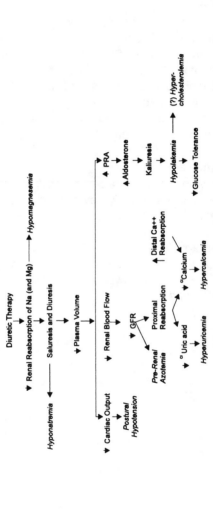

A pathogenic scheme for the various side effects of diuretics. (From Kaplan NM. *Clinical Hypertension*, 7th ed., Baltimore, MD: Williams & Wilkins, 1998.)

TABLE 13.1

Characteristics of Diuretics

Drug	Daily Dosage, mg	Duration of Action, h
Thiazides		
Bendroflumethiazide (Naturetin)	2.5-5.0	18
Benzthiazide (Exna)	12.5-50	12-18
Chlorothiazide (Diuril)	125-500	6-12
Cyclothiazide (Anhydron)	0.5-2.0	18-24
Hydrochlorothiazide (Esidrix, HydroDIURIL, Microzide)	12.5-50	12-18
Hydroflumethiazide (Saluron, Diucardin)	12.5-50	18-24
Methylclothiazide (Enduron, Aquatensen)	2.5-5.0	24
Polythiazide (Renese)	1.0-4.0	24-48
Trichlormethiazide (Metahydrin, Naqua)	1.0-4.0	24
Related sulfonamide compounds		
Chlorthalidone (Hygroton, Thalitone)	12.5-50	24-72
Indapamide (Lozol)	1.25-2.5	24

Metolazone	0.5-1.0	24
Mykrox	2.5-10	24
Zaroxolyn	25-100	18-24
Quinethazone (Hydromox)		
Loop diuretics		
Bumetanide (Bumex)	0.5-5.0	4-6
Ethacrynic acid (Edecrin)*	25-100	12
Furosemide (Lasix)	20-480	4-6
Torsemide (Demadex)	5-40	12
Potassium-sparing agents		
Amiloride (Midamor)	5-10	24
Eplerenone (Inspra)	50-400	24
Spironolactone (Aldactone)	25-100	8-12
Triamterene (Dyrenium)	50-150	12

Ethacrynic acid is the only nonsulfonamide diuretic for those who are intolerant of sulfa drugs.

TABLE 13.2

Effects of Varying Doses of Diuretics on Blood Pressure, Blood Chemistries, and Lipids

Changes from 0 to 10 weeks	Dose of Bendrofluazide (mg/day)				
	0	1.25	2.5	5.0	10.0
Blood Pressure (mm Hg)	-3/3	-13/10	-14/11	-13/10	-17/11
Potassium (mmol/L)	+0.09	-0.16	-0.20	-0.33	-0.45
Glucose (mg/dl)	-1.4	-3.4	+2.5	+0.7	+4.9
Cholesterol (mg/dl)	-2.2	-1.1	0.00	+4.6	+9.5

(From Carlsen et al.: Br Med J 1990;300:975)

References

Bennet WM, Porter GA: Efficacy and safety of metolazone in renal failure and the nephrotic syndrome. *J Clin Pharmacol* 1973;13:357–364.

Brater DC: Pharmacology of diuretics. *Am J Med Sci* 2000; 319:38–50.

Carlsen JE, Kober L, Torp-Pedersen C, Johansen P: Relation between dose of bendrofluazide, antihypertensive effect, and adverse biochemical effects. *Br Med J* 1990;300:975–978.

Flack JM, Cushman WC: Evidence for the efficacy of low-dose diuretic monotherapy. *Am J Med* 1996;101:53S–60S.

Franse LV, Pahor M, DiBari M, et al.: Hypokalemia associated with diuretic use and cardiovascular events in the systolic hypertension in the elderly program. *Hypertension* 2000;35: 611–616.

Frishman WH, Bryzinski BS, Coulson LR, et al.: A multifactorial trial design to assess combination therapy in hypertension. *Arch Intern Med* 1994;154:1461–1468.

Kasiske BL, Ma JZ, Kalil RSN, Louis TA: Effect of antihypertensive therapy on serum lipids. *Ann Intern Med* 1995;122: 133–141.

Lithell HO: Hyperinsulinemia, insulin resistance, and the treatment of hypertension. *Am J Hypertens* 1996;9:150S–154S.

Siscovick DS, Raghunathan TE, Psaty BM, et al.: Diuretic therapy for hypertension and the risk of primary cardiac arrest. *N Engl J Med* 1994;330:1852–1857.

Weinberger MH, Roniker B, Krause SL, Weiss RJ. Eplerenone, a selective aldosterone blocker, in mild-to-moderate hypertension. *Am J Hypertens* 2002;15:709–716.

Whang R, Flink EB, Dyckner T, Wester PO, Aikawa JK, Ryan MP: Magnesium depletion as a cause of refractory potassium repletion. *Arch Intern Med* 1985;145:1585–1589.

Wilcox CS: Metabolic and adverse effects of diuretics. *Semin Nephrol* 1999;19:557–568.

NOTES

#14 Diuretics: Loop and K⁺ Sparers

Loop Diuretics
Potassium-Sparing Agents

Some hypertensive patients may require more potent diuretics than thiazides. Those who receive thiazides may be protected from potassium wastage by the concomitant use of potassium-sparing agents.

LOOP DIURETICS

Loop diuretics exert a maximal natriuretic effect of 20 percent of the filtered load, some three to four times more than the thiazide diuretics, by blocking $NaCl$ reabsorption in the thick ascending limb of the loop of Henle. These agents must enter the tubular fluid to work. Therefore, when renal blood flow is reduced, larger doses are needed. Their entry into the tubule may be competitively blocked by organic acids and drugs such as probenecid.

Loop diuretics are primarily indicated for patients with reduced renal function (serum creatinine above 2.0 mg/dl) wherein thiazides are ineffectual or when there is a need for more potent diuretics, as with minoxidil therapy.

The two agents most widely used, furosemide (Lasix) and burmetanide (Bumex), are short-acting, with their effects lasting three to six hours. These must be given two or three times per day to maintain the slight shrinkage of plasma volume needed to keep BP down. A longer-acting loop diuretic, torsemide (Demadex), may provide

14.

a sustained antihypertensive effect with one or two doses per day.

Another loop diuretic, ethacrynic acid (Ede-crin), is little used because of its greater ototoxic-ity, except in those intolerant to sulfa drugs.

Side effects are similar to those seen with thi-azides, with the exception of hypercalcemia. These drugs will cause less severe biochemical changes because of their shorter durations of action.

POTASSIUM-SPARING AGENTS

Four potassium-sparing agents are now available: two, aldosterone antagonists, and the other two, inhibitors of tubular potassium (K^+) secretion. These agents are helpful in:
- Reducing thiazide-induced K^+ wastage
- Specifically treating hyperaldosteronism

Spironolactone (Aldactone) + HCT = Aldactazide; Eplerenone (Inspra)

Spironolactone competitively blocks the uptake of aldosterone by its receptors, thereby antagonizing its actions. It will reduce diuretic-induced K^+ loss. However, its major use is in treat-ment of states of aldosterone excess, whether primary or secondary (e.g., cirrhosis with ascites). Only 25 to 50 mg per day is needed for reduction in K^+ loss, but more may be needed to block hyperaldosteronism. In experimental ani-mals, spironolactone will inhibit myocardial fibro-sis, and it has been shown to reduce mortality in patients with congestive heart failure (CHF).

Side effects include:

- A capability to induce hyperkalemia, particularly when given in combination with an ACEI or an ARB to elderly, diabetic, or renal patients.
- Possible interference with testosterone synthesis, leading to impotence and gynecomastia in men and mastodynia in women.

A more specific aldosterone antagonist, eplerenone, has been approved.

Triamterene (Dyrenium) + HCT = Dyazide or Maxzide

Triamterene is the K^+ sparer contained in combination with HCT. It is sold in the United States as Dyazide or Maxzide.

For most patients with mild hypertension, one-half the smaller dose containing 25 mg of HCT should be used (12.5 mg of HCT).

Side effects are rare. Hyperkalemia is rarely seen except in patients with renal insufficiency who are also given potassium. Renal tubular damage and renal stones have been reported.

Amiloride (Midamor) + HCT = Moduretic

Amiloride is chemically distinct and acts differently than triamterene. However, the effects of these two K^+ sparers are quite similar. They both have limited natriuretic effects but inhibit K^+ secretion in the collecting duct. Moduretic also has 50 mg of HCT; one-half a tablet may be adequate for most patients.

References

Andersson P-O, H-Andersen H, Hagman A, Henning R: Potassium sparing by amiloride during thiazide therapy in hypertension. *Clin Pharmacol Ther* 1984;36:197–200.

Dunn CJ, Fitton A, Brogden RN: Torasemide: An update of its pharmacological properties and therapeutic efficacy. *Drugs* 1995;49:121–142.

Ellison DH: The physiologic basis of diuretic synergism: Its role in treating diuretic resistance. *Ann Intern Med* 1991;114: 886–895.

Funder JW: Non-genomic actions of aldosterone: Role in hypertension. *Curr Opin Nephrol Hypertens* 2001;10:227–230.

Hutcheon DE, Martinez JC: A decade of development in diuretic drug therapy. *J Clin Pharmacol* 1986;26:567–579.

Pitt B, Zannad F, Remme WJ, et al.: The effect of spironolactone on morbidity and mortality in patients with severe heart failure. *N Engl J Med* 1999;341:709–717.

Rose BD: Diuretics. *Kidney Int* 1991;39:336–352.

Schepkens H, Vanholder R, Billiouw J-M, Lameire N: Life-threatening hyperkalemia during combined therapy with angiotensin-converting enzyme inhibitors and spironolactone: An analysis of 25 cases. *Am J Med* 2001;110:438–441.

Spence JD, Wong DG, Lindsay RM: Effects of triameterene and amiloride on urinary sediment in hypertensive patients taking hydrochlorothiazide. *Lancet* 1985;2:73–75.

Weber KT, Sun Y, Guarda E: Structural remodeling in hypertensive heart disease and the role of hormones. *Hypertension* 1994;23:869–877.

Weinberger MH, Roniker B, Krause SL, Weiss RJ. Eplerenone, a selective aldosterone blocker, in mild-to-moderate hypertension. *Am J Hypertens* 2002;15:709–716.

Wollam GL, Tarazi RC, Bravo EL, Dustan HP: Diuretic potency of combined hydrochlorothiazide and furosemide therapy in patients with azotemia. *Am J Med* 1982;72:939–937.

#15 Adrenergic Inhibitors: Peripheral

Reserpine
Guanethidine
Guanadrel

The second major class of drugs includes those that inhibit the activity of the adrenergic (sympathetic) nervous system. As shown in Table 15.1, the primary sites of action vary from the brain to the peripheral neurons. Some act as competitive inhibitors of alpha-receptors and others as blockers of beta-receptors.

The peripheral-acting agents are shown to include reserpine, which acts in the CNS as well as on peripheral neurons. These drugs were among the first used antihypertensives but are now much less used as other agents have become available. Reserpine remains an effective, generally safe, inexpensive, once-a-day drug that works well, particularly in combination with a diuretic.

RESERPINE (Serpasil)

Reserpine, an ingredient of Indian snakeroot, acts by decreasing the transport of norepinephrine (NE) into its storage granules within the adrenergic nerve endings, thereby depleting the amount of the neurotransmitter available when the nerves are stimulated.

Small amounts are effective. When used with a diuretic, as little as 0.05 mg per day may be adequate. Larger doses of 0.25 mg are frequently used, either alone or in combination.

Side effects include:
• Nasal stuffiness

15.

- Sedation
- Mental depression

These side effects are lessened with smaller doses. Patients receiving the drug should be forewarned about symptoms of depression.

Claims that reserpine use was associated with an increased risk of breast cancer have not been documented and have been attributed to bias introduced by selected exclusion of certain patients from the original studies.

GUANETHIDINE (Ismelin)

Guanethidine was a popular agent, since it could be used once a day in patients with all degrees of hypertension and caused no CNS side effects. The drug caused profound inhibition of peripheral sympathetic nervous activity by blocking the exit of NE from its storage granules, frequently leading to:
- Postural hypotension
- Diarrhea
- Failure of ejaculation

Although the drug can be well tolerated with careful titration and avoidance of rapid postural changes, the drug has largely been relegated to a last-option status.

GUANADREL (Hylorel)

Guanadrel, a guanethidine-like agent, is easier to use than guanethidine because of its shorter duration of action and less sustained interference with peripheral adrenergic action.

Side effects are similar to guanethidine but less common. The antihypertensive efficacy is comparable to that of methyldopa.

Characteristics of
Adrenergic Inhibitors

TABLE 15.1

Drug	Trade Name	Dose Range (mg/day)	Side Effects
Peripheral			
Reserpine	Serpasil	0.05 to 0.25	Sedation, nasal congestion, depression
Guanethidine	Ismelin	10 to 150	Orthostatic hypotension, diarrhea
Guanadrel	Hylorel	10 to 75	Orthostatic hypotension
Central			
Methyldopa	Aldomet	500 to 3,000	Sedation, liver dysfunction, fever, "autoimmune" disorders
Clonidine	Catapres	0.2 to 1.2	Sedation, dry mouth, "withdrawal hypertension"
Guanabenz	Wytensin	8 to 64	Sedation, dry mouth, dizziness
Guanfacine	Tenex	1 to 3	(Same as Guanabenz)
Alpha-Blockers			
Doxazosin	Cardura	1 to 16	Postural hypotension, fatigue, sedation
Prazosin	Minipress	2 to 20	(Same as Doxazosin)
Terazosin	Hytrin	1 to 20	(Same as Doxazosin)

Beta-Blockers		Serious: bronchospasm, congestive heart failure, masking of insulin-induced hypoglycemia, depression
Acebutolol	Sectral	200 to 800
Atenolol	Tenormin	25 to 100
Betaxolol	Kerlone	5 to 20
Bisoprolol	Zebeta	2.5 to 10
Carteolol	Cartrol	2.5 to 10
Metoprolol	Lopressor	50 to 300
Nadolol	Corgard	40 to 320
Penbutolol	Levatol	10 to 20
Pindolol	Visken	10 to 60
Propanolol	Inderal	40 to 480
Timolol	Blocadren	20 to 60
		Others: poor peripheral circulation, insomnia, bradycardia, fatigue, decreased exercise tolerance, hypertriglyceridemia, decreased HDL-cholesterol
Combined Alpha- and Beta-Blockers		
Labetalol	Normodyne, Trandate	200 to 1,200	Postural hypotension, beta-blocking side effects
Carvedilol	Coreg	12.5 to 50	(Same as Labetalol)

References

Finnerty FA, Brogden RN: Guanadrel: A review of its pharmacodynamic and pharmacokinetic properties and therapeutic use in hypertension. *Drugs* 1985;30:22–31.

Fraser HS: Reserpine: A tragic victim of myths, marketing, and fashionable prescribing. *Clin Pharmacol Ther* 1996;60:368–373.

Horwitz RI, Feinstein AR: Exclusion bias and the false relationship of reserpine and breast cancer. *Arch Intern Med* 1985;145:1873–1875.

Krönig B, Pittrow DB, Kirch W, et al.: Different concepts in first-line treatment of essential hypertension. *Hypertension* 1997; 29:651–658.

Lederle FA, Applegate WB, Grimm RH Jr.: Reserpine and the medical market place. *Arch Intern Med* 1993;153:705–706.

NOTES

115

#16 Adrenergic Inhibitors:
Central Agonists

Methyldopa
Clonidine
Guanabenz
Guanfacine

Central agonists act as alpha$_2$-receptor agonists, primarily on vasomotor centers within the brain, thereby decreasing the sympathetic outflow from the CNS (Figure 16.1). As a result, cardiac output is decreased slightly, but the main hemodynamic effect is a fall in peripheral vascular resistance.

Although the four currently available members of this group differ in some ways, they share common mechanisms of action and side effects, mainly sedation and dry mouth. Methyldopa, however, has some unique "autoimmune" side effects.

METHYLDOPA (Aldomet)

Mechanism of Action

Once the most popular drug after thiazide diuretics, methyldopa is now rarely used, since newer agents have become available that are equally effective and better tolerated. Its major current use is in the treatment of hypertension during pregnancy, since long experience has shown it not to harm the fetus.

Methyldopa is converted into alpha-methyl-norepinephrine, which acts as an agonist (stimulant) of central alpha-receptors. This leads to a decrease in discharge from central vasomotor

16.

centers, damping sympathetic nervous activity throughout the body.

Dosage

To reduce the impact of the centrally mediated side effects (sedation and dry mouth, in particular), the initial dose should be no more than 250 mg twice per day. The total dosage can be raised to 3 g per day; however, 1 g twice per day will do almost all that is possible with the drug.

Side Effects

Beyond the common side effects of sedation and dry mouth, many patients experience a more subtle decrease in mental alertness. These side effects are common to all four central alpha-agonists. Methyldopa, however, induces a number of "autoimmune" disorders, including:

- Positive Coombs tests in as many as 25 percent and hemolytic anemia, very rarely
- Abnormal liver function tests in eight percent
- Severe hepatic necrosis in a small number
- Attack upon virtually every other organ, though frequency is quite low

These immune-inflammatory processes are not seen with other central agonists that are equal in effectiveness. Therefore, continued use of methyldopa is difficult to justify and must be attributed to hard-to-change prescribing habits.

CLONIDINE (Catapres)

Clonidine, similar to methyldopa, differs in two important ways:

- Its duration of action is shorter
- Its dosage is smaller so that it can be absorbed through the skin

Dosage

The starting dose should be 0.1 mg two or three times per day. The small quantity of drug needed to exert the antihypertensive effect has also been placed in a patch for transdermal absorption, thereby providing up to seven days of therapy. The patch may provide smoother control of hypertension with fewer side effects.

Side Effects

When the drug is stopped, sympathetic nervous activity may bounce back rather quickly from its suppressed state and may overshoot, inducing rebound hypertension. This problem is infrequent when the total dosage is kept below 0.8 mg per day and should be treated by reinstitution of therapy.

Local skin reactions may preclude use of the transdermal patch in 20 percent or more of patients.

GUANABENZ (Wytensin)

Guanabenz is an attractive central alpha-agonist for two reasons:
- It lowers total serum cholesterol levels by five to 10 percent
- It causes little reactive fluid retention

The drug mimics the mode of action and side effects of clonidine in most ways.

The starting dosage should be 4 mg twice per day, and the maximum dosage can reach a total of 64 mg per day.

GUANFACINE (Tenex)

Guanfacine is also similar to clonidine, although it causes less somnolence and propensity to the withdrawal syndrome.

Dosage is 1 to 3 mg once per day. As a once-a-day preparation, guanfacine is the most attractive of the alpha$_2$-agonists.

NEWER AGENTS

Although not now available in the United States, drugs that also stimulate central imidazoline receptors (e.g., moxonidine and rilmenidine) are being used elsewhere with claims of lesser CNS sedative effects than the alpha$_2$-agonists.

FIGURE 16.1

Mode of Action of Central Alpha$_2$-Agonists

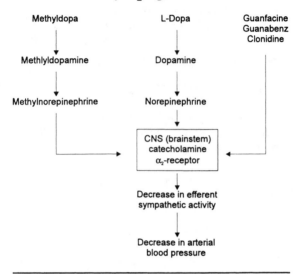

Schematic representation of the common mechanism underlying the hypotensive actions of methyldopa, clonidine, and guanabenz. (From Henning M. In: vanZwieten PA (ed.) Handbook of Hypertensin, Vol. 3, Amsterdam: Elsevier Science Publishers, 1984.)

References

Clobass Study Group. Low-dose clonidine administration in the treatment of mild or moderate essential hypertension: Results from a double-blind placebo-controlled study (Clobass). *J Hypertens* 1990;8:539–546.

Holmes B, Brogden RN, Heel RC, Speight TM, Avery GS: Guanabenz: A review of its pharmacodynamic properties and therapeutic efficacy in hypertension. *Drugs* 1983;26:212–229.

Kelton JG: Impaired reticuloendothelial function in patients treated with methyldopa. *N Engl J Med* 1985;313:596–600.

Lewin A, Alderman MH, Mathur P: Antihypertensive efficacy of guanfacine and prazosin in patients with mild to moderate essential hypertension. *J Clin Pharmacol* 1990;30:1081–1087.

Schmidt GR, Schuna AA, Goodfriend TL: Transdermal clonidine compared with hydrochlorothiazide as monotherapy in elderly hypertensive males. *J Clin Pharmacol* 1989;39:133–139.

van Zwieten PA: The renaissance of centrally acting antihypertensive drugs. *J Hypertens* 1999;17(Suppl 3):S15–S21.

#17 Adrenergic Inhibitors: Alpha-Blockers

Alpha$_1$-blockers currently available are:
- Doxazosin (Cardura)
- Prazosin (Minipress)
- Terazosin (Hytrin)

Mode of Action

Alpha-blockers have a much higher affinity for the post-synaptic alpha$_1$-receptors located on the vascular smooth muscle cells than on the presynaptic alpha$_2$-receptors located on the neuronal membrane. Blockade of the alpha$_1$-receptors inhibits the uptake of catecholamines by the smooth muscle cells, thereby blunting vasoconstriction and inducing peripheral vasodilation (see Figure 17.1).

The minimal blockage of alpha$_2$-receptors on the neuron leaves them open to the effects of catecholamines present within the synaptic cleft, thereby inhibiting the release of additional NE from the neuronal storage granules. The nonselective alpha-blockers (phentolamine [Regitine] and phenoxybenzamine [Dibenzyline]), which also block the neuronal alpha$_2$-receptors, remove the inhibitory effect upon NE release so that more NE enters the circulation, blunting the antihypertensive effect and causing tachycardia. The latter drugs are only useful for therapy of pheochromocytoma.

Dosage

The initial dose of alpha-blockers may lower BP excessively, particularly in those already taking diuretics. First-dose hypotension can be obviated by:

- Stopping the diuretic for two days before beginning treatment with alpha-blockers
- Giving only 1 mg of the drug
- Warning patients about the possibility of postural symptoms

Although some suggest that patients take the first dose at bedtime, to preclude trouble if patients arise from bed during the night, the first dose may be taken on a day when patients can lie around and better manage postural symptoms. In fact, the problem is very infrequent, particularly with the slower-acting doxazosin and terazosin.

Dosage should be slowly increased to a maximum of 20 mg per day. Prazosin should be taken twice or three times per day, whereas doxazosin and terazosin can be taken once daily.

Side Effects

Beyond the very rare first-dose hypotension, some patients continue to experience dizziness and a few note tachycardia or GI distress. Alpha-blockers rarely cause CNS side effects such as sedation or dry mouth.

The alpha-blocker (doxazosin) arm of the ALLHAT trial was discontinued because of a higher incidence of heart failure compared to that seen with the diuretic (chlorthalidone). Since mortality rates were identical, the heart failure must have been mild and likely the consequence of rather abrupt discontinuation of diuretic and ACEI therapy in high-risk patients who were then started on a low dose (1 mg) of the alpha-blocker. This problem should rarely, if ever, arise in clinical practice.

Lipid and Metabolic Effects

Beta-blockers often raise serum triglycerides and lower HDL-cholesterol levels (see Section #18). Alpha-blockers appear to do the opposite; in many patients:

- Total cholesterol and triglyceride levels are lowered
- HDL-cholesterol is raised

Selective alpha$_1$-receptor blockers are particularly useful in young patients who wish to remain physically active. In such patients, the use of beta-blockers often reduces exercise capacity by lowering cardiac output.

Alpha-blockers provide good antihypertensive effects without worsening lipids or lowering potassium, as do diuretics. Moreover, prazosin and doxazosin reduce plasma insulin levels and improve glucose tolerance.

Benign Prostatic Hypertrophy

Selective alpha$_1$-blockers relieve the obstructive symptoms of benign prostatic hypertrophy, apparently by relaxing the tone of prostatic muscle but perhaps by also reducing the mass of prostatic hypertrophy. They are now often the initial therapy for prostatism. Elderly men with prostatism and hypertension are obviously excellent candidates for such therapy.

FIGURE 17.1

Mode of Action of Alpha$_1$-Blockers

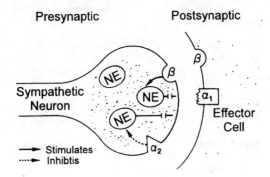

Prazosin Inhibits Postsynaptic α_1 Receptor
But Not Presynaptic α_2 Receptor

A schematic representation of a neuron and a vascular smooth muscle cell, showing how prazosin preferentially blocks the alpha$_1$-receptor and leaves the presynaptic alpha$_2$-receptor unblocked. (From Kaplan NM. *Clinical Hypertension* 7th ed., Baltimore: Williams & Wilkins, 1998.)

References

ALLHAT Officers and Coordinators for the ALLHAT Collaborative Research Group: Major cardiovascular events in hypertensive patients randomized to doxazosin vs chlorthalidone. *JAMA* 2000;283:1967–1975.

Andersson P-E, Lithell H: Metabolic effects of doxazosin and enalapril in hypertriglyceridemic, hypertensive men: Relationship to changes in skeletal muscle blood flow. *Am J Hypertens* 1996;9:323–333.

Khoury AF, Kaplan NM: Alpha-blocker therapy of hypertension: An unfulfilled promise. *JAMA* 1991;266:394–398.

Lepor H, Kaplan SA, Klimberg I, et al.: Doxazosin for benign prostatic hyperplasia: Long-term efficacy and safety in hypertensive and normotensive patients. *J Urol* 1997;157:525–530.

Levy D, Walmsley P, Levenstein M, et al.: Principal results of the hypertension and lipid trial (HALT): A multicenter study of doxazosin in patients with hypertension. *Am Heart J* 1996; 131:966–973.

Martell N, Luque M: Doxazosin added to single-drug therapy in hypertensive patients with benign prostatic hypertrophy. *J Clin Hypertens* 2001;3:218–223.

Rabkin SW, Huff MW, Newman C, Sim D, Carruthers SG: Lipids and lipoproteins during antihypertensive drug therapy: Comparison of doxazosin and atenolol in a randomized, double-blind trial. The Alpha Beta Canada Study. *Hypertension* 1994;24:241–248.

NOTES

#18 Adrenergic Inhibitors: Beta-Blockers

Beta-blockers, until recently, were the second most widely used drugs after diuretics. Recently their use has decreased for both practical and theoretical reasons: they cause some significant side effects and they do not relieve the peripheral vascular resistance that is the fundamental mechanism that sustains hypertension. Moreover, when used alone, they have not provided as much primary protection against coronary disease as other classes of drugs, particularly in the elderly. On the other hand, beta-blockers should be more frequently used in those with active coronary disease and/or survivors of a myocardial infarction (MI) where they provide excellent secondary protection.

Mode of Action

Beta-blockers without intrinsic sympathomimetic activity (ISA) lower BP by:
- Reducing cardiac output
- Inhibiting the release of renin
- Reducing NE release from neurons
- Decreasing central vasomotor activity

In the peripheral vessels, beta-blockade inhibits vasodilation acutely, but over time peripheral resistance usually returns to normal.

Beta-blockers with ISA (e.g., pindolol, acebutolol, and penbutolol) lower BP without reducing cardiac output and may decrease peripheral resistance by causing some sympathetic stimulation while blocking endogenous catechol effects. They cause less bradycardia and cold extremities.

18

Differences among Beta-Blockers

Beyond different degrees of ISA, beta-blockers differ in lipid solubility and relative selectivity in blocking beta$_1$-receptors in the heart vs. beta$_2$-receptors elsewhere (see Figure 18.1).

The more lipid soluble, the more of the drug that is taken up and metabolized on the first pass through the liver and the more of the drug that enters the brain. The greater hepatic uptake results in inactivation of the first few doses until uptake is saturated. A smaller IV dose may produce much greater effects than a larger oral dose. Lipid-soluble agents generally have shorter durations of action because of more rapid hepatic inactivation.

Comparable lipid solubility is:

Very soluble:
• Betaxolol
• Metoprolol
• Propranolol
• Timolol

Somewhat soluble:
• Acebutolol
• Bisoprolol
• Pindolol

Less soluble:
• Atenolol
• Carteolol
• Nadolol

Those that are less lipid soluble remain unmetabolized in the blood and are slowly excreted through the kidneys; therefore, their durations of action are longer, less of the drug enters the brain, and there may be fewer CNS side effects.

Beta-blockers that are more active on cardiac beta$_1$-receptors than on beta$_2$-receptors include:
- Acebutolol
- Atenolol
- Betaxolol
- Bisoprolol
- Metoprolol

This selectivity can be shown with acute administration of single doses. These agents cause less decrease in peripheral blood flow or pulmonary air movement than noncardioselective agents. However, none are truly cardioselective, and most differences disappear with chronic use or larger doses.

Clinical Effectiveness
The antihypertensive effectiveness of various beta-blockers in equivalent doses is similar. When used alone, beta-blockers are somewhat less effective in black and elderly patients. This difference may reflect lower plasma renin levels in elderly and black patients.

Beta-blockers may be particularly useful in patients with:
- Hypertension associated with tachycardia and high cardiac output

Hypertension accompanied by:
- Angina or prior MI
- Migraine
- Glaucoma
- Other coincidental diseases that are responsive to beta-blockade

Beta-blockers and diuretics were given preference for initial therapy in the US JNC-6 because they had been the only classes of drugs tested in large clinical trials shown to reduce mortality. Although beta-blockers have been shown to reduce recurrent MI and sudden death among patients who recently experienced acute MI, in only one of five large trials have they been found to reduce the incidence of initial MIs below that seen with diuretic-based therapy. In the Medical Research Council (MRC) trial in the elderly, atenolol gave no coronary protection, whereas a diuretic did.

A combination of bisoprolol and a low (6.25 mg) dose of hydrochlorothiazide (ZIAC) was approved for initial therapy of hypertension, after it was shown to provide equal efficacy but fewer side effects than larger doses of the two individual drugs.

SIDE EFFECTS

Beta-blockers may be associated with various side effects. Most are predictable in view of their pharmacological action. Some are more common in those agents that are noncardioselective or lipid soluble or that lack ISA.

Cardiac
Beta-blockers with little or no ISA induce bradycardia, which is usually asymptomatic and should be disregarded. Patients who monitor the degree of physical activity by heart rate should be made aware that maximal heart rate will be approximately 20 percent lower. The state of

physical conditioning can be achieved in the presence of beta-blockade, but reduced exercise ability and easier fatigue are often noted.

Beta-blockers tend to slow the rate of A-V conduction and may worsen the degree of heart block.

Pulmonary

Bronchospasm may result if patients are in need of beta-agonist effects to maintain patent airways. Allergic reactions may be more frequent and symptomatic.

Metabolic

Diabetics who take insulin and are prone to hypoglycemia should be given beta-blockers with great caution. The response to hypoglycemia largely depends on catecholamine stimulation of glucose synthesis and release, particularly in insulin-dependent diabetics who are also unable to secrete glucagon. Insulin-induced hypoglycemia may be longer in duration and more severe in the presence of a beta-blocker. Beta-blockers mask the usual symptoms of hypoglycemia, such as tremor, tachycardia, and hunger. Sweating, however, is not diminished, and diabetics given beta-blockers should be aware of the significance of sweating as a warning signal.

Hypertriglyceridemia and a concomitant fall in HDL-cholesterol are common with beta-blockers, though less marked with those having high degrees of ISA. Serum triglyceride levels rise an average of 30 percent with most beta-blockers.

The insulin resistance and hyperinsulinemia present in hypertension may be further aggravated by beta-blockers, and an increased incidence of diabetes has been reported with their use.

Central

Fatigue is common and may be related to the decreased cardiac output seen with non-ISA beta-blockers or to central effects. Bad dreams, even hallucinations, may be noted. Claims for increased incidence of depression have not been substantiated. These effects are less common with the lipid-insoluble agents and in those patients with ISA.

Renal

A 10- to 20-percent fall in renal blood flow and GFR has been noted with most beta-blockers. The effect may reflect renal vasoconstriction. Fluid retention has been noted in a small number of low-renin hypertensive patients given propranolol.

OVERVIEW OF THERAPY

In the past 25 years, beta-blockers have been widely used as the first or second drug in the treatment of hypertension. They are effective and usually well tolerated. Their effectiveness is increased by low doses of a diuretic. However, they may cause fatigue and loss of exercise ability. Of more concern are the lipid and glucose-insulin abnormalities seen with those beta-blockers that lack ISA.

These drugs protect against recurrent MIs but have not been shown in most studies to protect against a first heart attack. However, atenolol reduced cardiovascular mortality when given to patients with coronary disease who underwent noncardiac surgery. Moreover, beta-blockers have been found to improve survival rates after acute MI with left ventricular dysfunction and provide hemodynamic benefits for patients with congestive failure.

FIGURE 18.1

Classification of Beta-Blockers

Beta-Adrenoceptor Blocking Drugs

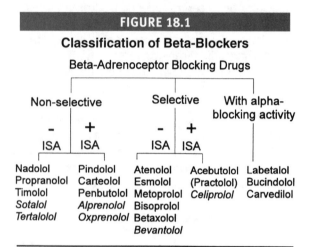

Non-selective		Selective		With alpha-blocking activity
– ISA	+ ISA	– ISA	+ ISA	
Nadolol	Pindolol	Atenolol	Acebutolol	Labetalol
Propranolol	Carteolol	Esmolol	(Practolol)	Bucindolol
Timolol	Penbutolol	Metoprolol	*Celiprolol*	Carvedilol
Sotalol	*Alprenolol*	Bisoprolol		
Tertalolol	*Oxprenolol*	Betaxolol		
		Bevantolol		

Classification of beta-adrenoceptor blockers based on cardioselectivity and intrinsic sympathomimetic activity (ISA). (Those not approved for use in the U.S. are in italics.)

References

Abraham WT: β-blockers: The new standard therapy for mild heart failure. *Arch Intern Med* 2000;160:1237–1247.

Christensen KL, Mulvany MJ: Vasodilatation, not hypotension, improves resistance vessel design during treatment of essential hypertension: A literature survey. *J Hypertens* 2001;19:1001–1006.

Frishman WH, Bryzinski BS, Coulson LR, et al.: A multifactorial trial design to assess combination therapy in hypertension. *Arch Intern Med* 1994;154:1461–1468.

Goldstein S: β-blockers in hypertensive and coronary heart disease. *Arch Intern Med* 1996;156:1267–1276.

Gress TW, Nieto FJ, Shahar E, et al.: Hypertension and antihypertensive therapy as risk factors for type 2 diabetes mellitus. *N Engl J Med* 2000;342:905–912.

Lund-Johansen P, Omvik P: Acute and chronic hemodynamic effects of drugs with different actions on adrenergic receptors: A comparison between α-blockers and different types of β-blockers with and without vasodilating effect. *Cardiovasc Drugs Ther* 1991;5:605–616.

Mangano DT, Layug EL, Wallace A, et al.: Effect of atenolol on mortality and cardiovascular morbidity after noncardiac surgery. *N Eng J Med* 1996;334:1713–1720.

Morgan TO, Anderson AIE, MacInnis RJ: ACE inhibitors, beta-blockers, calcium blockers, and diuretics for the control of systolic hypertension. *Am J Hypertens* 2001;14:241–247.

MRC Working Party. Medical Research Council Trial of treatment of hypertension in older adults: Principal results. *Br Med J* 1992;304:405–412.

Perez-Stable EJ, Halliday R, Gardiner PS, et al.: The effects of propranolol on cognitive function and quality of life: A randomized trial among patients with diastolic hypertension. *Am J Med* 2000;108:359–365.

#19 Adrenergic Inhibitors: Combined Alpha- and Beta-Blockers

Until recently, labetalol (Normodyne, Trandate) was the only drug currently available with both alpha- and beta-blocking effects. Carvedilol (Coreg) has both beta-blocking and vasodilatory effects; thus, it is considered in the same class as labetalol. Nebivolol, not now available in the United States, is another vasodilating beta-blocker.

Mode of Action

In smaller doses, labetalol has three times more beta-blocking effects than alpha-blocking action. A maximal degree of alpha-blockade occurs with increasing doses, whereas the beta-blocking effects continue, so that the ratio increases to 6:1 or higher.

The beta-blocking action is similar to that seen with propranolol, which is noncardioselective and lipid soluble. The alpha-blocking effect is similar to that seen with prazosin, inducing peripheral vasodilation. As a result of the combination of effects, BP falls mainly from a decrease in peripheral resistance, with little effect on heart rate or cardiac output. The actions of carvedilol are similar: nonselective beta- and alpha-blocker effects.

When taken by mouth, carvedilol and labetalol should be given twice a day to ensure 24-hour efficacy. When labetalol is given IV, the antihypertensive effect is rapid and may be profound, with a propensity to postural hypotension if patients stand.

Dosage

19

With labetalol, 100 mg twice per day is usually an adequate starting dose, with a maximum of 2,400 mg per day. By vein, the drug may be given initially in a 20 mg dose by slow injection, with repeated 20 to 80 mg doses at 10-minute intervals. The maximal effect of each dose is usually seen within 10 minutes, and the duration of action is up to six hours. The drug may also be given by slow continuous infusion at an initial rate of 2 mg per minute, with 50 to 200 mg usually required for adequate response. Carvedilol can be started at 12.5 mg and the dosage raised to 50 mg twice a day.

Side Effects

Some side effects are related to alpha-blockade; these include:
- Postural dizziness
- Scalp tingling
- Nasal stuffiness

Other side effects are related to beta-blockade; these include:
- Fatigue
- Vivid dreams
- Bronchospasm
- Cold extremities
- Claudication

Rare instances of severe hepatotoxicity have been reported with labetalol.

These drugs cause less of a rise in serum triglycerides and less worsening of insulin sensitivity than do beta-blockers.

Clinical Use

Orally, labetalol should be used primarily for treatment of moderate to severe degrees of hypertension. IV, it should be useful in those who have need for rapid, though not instantaneous, reduction of markedly elevated BPs. Carvedilol has been found to be useful in the treatment of chronic heart failure, reducing morbidity and mortality when given to patients receiving digoxin, diuretics, and ACEIs.

References

Clark JA, Zimmerman HJ, Tanner LA: Labetalol hepatotoxicity. *Ann Intern Med* 1990;113:210–213.

Lebel M, et al.: Labetalol infusion in hypertensive emergencies. *Clin Pharmacol Ther* 1985;37:615–618.

Lithell H, Andersson P-E: Metabolic effects of carvedilol in hypertensive patients. *Eur J Clin Pharmacol* 1997;52:13–17.

Packer M, Bristow MR, Cohn JN, et al.: The effect of carvedilol on morbidity and mortality in patients with chronic heart failure. *N Engl J Med* 1996;334:1349–1355.

Strangaard S, Paulson OB: Antihypertensive drugs and cerebral circulation. *Eur J Clin Invest* 1996;26:625–630.

Townsend RR, DiPette DJ, Goodman R, et al.: Combined α/β-blockade vs β-1 selective blockade in essential hypertension in black and white patients. *Clin Pharmacol Ther* 1990;48:665–675.

Tzemos N, Lim PO, MacDonald TM: Nebivolol reverses endothelial dysfunction in essential hypertension: A randomized, double-blind, crossover study. *Circulation* 2001;104:511–514.

#20 Vasodilators: Direct-Acting

These agents are used less now that other vasodilating drugs are available, including ACEIs, ARBs, and CCBs. These newer agents have fewer adverse effects, but the older drugs are much less expensive and equally effective.

Other direct vasodilators, including nitric oxide donors, are under investigation.

Minoxidil is now known to act as an opener of potassium channels. A large number of such agents are under investigation. One, pinacidil, is available elsewhere but is not approved for use in the United States.

The use of direct-acting vasodilators has been made practical by combining them with diuretics and adrenergic inhibitors. Large doses of hydralazine and minoxidil have been used as part of triple therapy to treat severe degrees of hypertension.

These drugs alone induce significant dilation of resistance arterioles with a fall in peripheral resistance. The resultant fall in BP activates baroreceptors that set off sympathetic reflexes, causing:

- Release of both renin and catecholamines
- Stimulation of the heart
- Constriction of veins

The fall in BP also leads to renal retention of sodium, expanding fluid volume.

Various side effects are seen as a result of all these compensatory reactions to the vasodilator-induced fall in BP including:

- Tachycardia
- Flushing

- Headaches
- A loss of antihypertensive efficacy

With concomitant use of an adrenergic inhibitor and a diuretic, various compensatory reactions are inhibited and BP falls even more, thus reducing side effects. A beta-blocker is usually used as the adrenergic inhibitor, and a thiazide is usually chosen as the diuretic; but furosemide or metolazone may be needed in patients with marked responses to minoxidil, particularly if they start with some degree of renal insufficiency.

20.

Clinical Use
In the past, hydralazine was often chosen as the third drug for those not responding adequately to a diuretic and an adrenergic inhibitor. The initial dose is usually 25 mg twice per day and may be increased to 200 mg twice per day, although total daily doses beyond 200 mg are associated with an increasing likelihood of a lupus-like reaction. Parenteral hydralazine is the preferred treatment for severe hypertension during pregnancy.

Minoxidil is often used for patients with severe hypertension, particularly when renal insufficiency is present. It can be given once per day, with total dosage from 5 to 60 mg. Its use is complicated by a marked tendency for:

- Fluid retention, requiring use of potent diuretics
- Hirsutism, precluding use of the drug in many women unwilling to have hair on their faces and elsewhere. Men are rarely concerned, and the drug is now available for use as topical treatment to regrow hair.

Side Effects

Most side effects are attributable to the activation of compensatory mechanisms to direct vasodilation, including:

- Tachycardia
- Flushing
- Headache

However, hydralazine also can cause a lupus-like reaction with:

- Fever
- Rash
- Arthralgias

Renal or CNS involvement is rare. The reaction is usually benign and disappears when the drug is stopped. Perry et al. found that patients who have reactions have no residual damage and a 10- to 15-year survival rate greater than similar patients who have not had reactions.

The tendency for fluid retention and hirsutism with minoxidil reflects its marked vasodilation of renal and skin arterioles.

Overview

Direct vasodilators are effective and generally well tolerated. However, their use has been receding in the face of equally effective ACEIs, ARBs, and CCBs that tend to cause fewer side effects.

Vasodilators that act via openings of vascular potassium channels are under clinical investigation. In addition, nitrates have been used as anti-hypertensives and other, longer-acting nitric oxide donors are under investigation.

References

Nielsen-Kudsk JE, Boesgaard S, Aldershvile J: K⁺ channel opening. *Heart* 1996;76:109–116.

Paterson-Brown S, Robson SC, Redfern N, et al.: Hydralazine boluses for the treatment of severe hypertension in pre-eclampsia. *Br J Obstet Gynaecol* 1994;101:409–413.

Perry HM Jr., Camel GH, Carmody SE, et al.: Survival in hydralazine-treated hypertensive patients with and without late toxicity. *J Chronic Dis* 1997;30:519–528.

Pontremoli R, Robaudo C, Gaiter A, et al.: Long-term minoxidil treatment in refractory hypertension and renal failure. *Clin Nephrol* 1991;35:39–43.

van Bortel LM, Spek JJ, Balkestein EJ, et al.: Is it possible to develop drugs that act more selectively on large arteries? *J Hypertens* 1999;17:701–705.

#21 Vasodilators: Calcium Channel Blockers

The CCBs now available are listed in Table 21.1. Amlodipine and felodipine are second-generation CCBs that offer even greater vasoselectivity than the others. A number of other CCBs, most of which are dihydropyridines similar to nifedipine, are under investigation. Mibefradil, a novel CCB that selectively blocks the T-type calcium channel, was approved but withdrawn because of multiple drug interactions.

Mode of Action

All CCBs lower BP by blocking calcium entry into vascular smooth muscle cells. The decrease in free intracellular calcium reduces vascular tone and contractility. Peripheral resistance and BP fall.

Diltiazem and verapamil also act within the S-A and A-V nodes, making them useful for the treatment of certain arrhythmias but adding to their interactions with beta-blockers to induce serious A-V conduction block.

Dihydropyridines, such as amlodipine and nifedipine, have no effect on sinus or A-V nodal conduction. This is an advantage in reducing beta-blocker interactions and a disadvantage in allowing for some reflex tachycardia.

Clinical Use

Most vasodilators were originally available in fairly short-acting formulations that require three doses per day for a sustained 24-hour antihypertensive effect. Now some (e.g., diltiazem, nifedipine, verapamil) are available in slow-release formulations; others (e.g., amlodipine) are inherently so long-acting that effects persist even for 48 hours. These drugs have been found by some to work better in older patients than younger patients and to work particularly well in blacks. They also work well in the face of high sodium intake irrespective of the degree of sodium sensitivity, and their effectiveness is enhanced by concomitant diuretics.

21

Long-acting dihydropyridines (nifedipine, nitrendipine) have reduced overall and stroke morbidity and mortality in three placebo-controlled trials in elderly hypertensives: the nonrandomized Shanghai Trial of Nifedipine in the Elderly (STONE) (Gong et al., 1996) and the randomized Systolic hypertension in Europe (SYST-EUR) trial (Staessen et al., 1997) and Systolic hypertension in China (SYST-CHINA) trial (Wang et al., 1999).

Liquid nifedipine, given either sublingually or swallowed, lowers BP markedly within 20 minutes. The profound fall in BP, which cannot be titrated, may induce cerebral or myocardial ischemia; thus, short-acting nifedipine should only be used when no other therapies are available and rapid reduction of BP is needed.

Although large doses of short-acting nifedipine were found to increase mortality after acute MI, the longer-acting CCBs have been shown in multiple large randomized controlled trials, when compared against either placebo or other active drugs, to provide excellent protection against coronary disease, strokes, and overall mortality.

Side Effects

The nature and severity of side effects differ considerably among the drugs (see Table 21.1).

The edema seen with dihydropyridines is localized to the ankles or legs, likely secondary to vasodilation. It may be so cosmetically bothersome as to preclude the use of these drugs.

Verapamil is most likely to cause A-V nodal dysfunction; thus, it should be used with great caution in combination with beta-blockers.

Although the secretion of most hormones is dependent on local release of calcium, hormonal secretions are affected very little by these drugs, and they may be safely used in diabetics. Short-term reductions in proteinuria have been seen with verapamil and diltiazem; the long-term effects of calcium blockers on renal function have not been adequately studied, but they are generally recommended only as additions to ACEIs and diuretics in order to achieve adequate control of hypertension.

CCBs are generally neutral in their effects on insulin sensitivity. They are similarly neutral in their effects on lipids.

Putative Serious Dangers of CCBs

A series of uncontrolled retrospective case-control studies purported to show an increase in coronary disease, GI bleeding, and cancer in patients given various short-acting CCBs. Subsequent prospective cohort, case-control studies, and randomized controlled trials (RCTs), with the currently available long-acting CCBs have found no such associations. In particular, felodipine was the initial therapy in the Hypertension Optimal Therapy (HOT) trial, and nifedipine and nitrendipine were the initial therapies in the three trials in the elderly, all of which found excellent coronary and stroke protection with no increase in cancer or

GI bleeding. Thus, the putative dangers of short-acting CCBs do not seem to apply to long-acting CCBs.

Overview

CCBs are effective antihypertensives in virtually all types of patients and have few contraindications. They will continue to be widely used with the availability of more vasoselective and longer-acting preparations. The ability to reduce BP (particularly well in elderly patients), the lack of interference from NSAIDs or high sodium intake, and the antianginal effects have led to widespread use of CCBs as antihypertensive agents.

TABLE 21.1

Characteristics of Calcium Channel Blockers (CCBs)

Drug	Trade Name	Usual Dose Range, Total mg/day (frequency per day)	Selected Side Effects and Comments
Nondihydropyridines			
Diltiazem	Cardizem SR	120-480 (2)	Conduction defects, nausea, headache
	Cardizem CD, Dilacor XL, Tiazac	120-480 (1)	
Verapamil	Isoptin SR, Calan SR	90-480 (2)	Constipation
	Verelan, Covera HS	120-480 (1)	
Dihydropyridines			
Amlodipine	Norvasc	2.5-10 (1)	Ankle edema, flushing, headache, gingival hyperplasia
Felodipine	Plendil	2.5-20 (1)	
Isradipine	DynaCirc, DynaCirc CR	5-20 (2,1)	
Nicardipine	Cardene SR	60-120 (2)	
Nifedipine	Procardia XL, Adalat CC	30-120 (1)	
Nisoldipine	Sular	20-40 (1)	

References

Abernathy DR, Schwartz JB: Calcium-antagonist drugs. *N Engl J Med* 1999;341:1447–1457.

Ad Hoc Subcommittee. Effects of calcium antagonist on the risks of coronary heart disease, cancer, and bleeding. *J Hypertens* 1997;15:105–115.

Alderman MH, Cohen H, Roqué R, Madhavan S: Effect of long-acting and short-acting calcium antagonists on cardiovascular outcomes in hypertensive patients. *Lancet* 1997;349:594–598.

Blood Pressure Lowering Treatment Trialists' Collaboration: Effects of ACE inhibitors, calcium antagonists, and other blood-pressure-lowering drugs: Results of prospectively designed overviews of randomised trials. *Lancet* 2000;355:1955–1964.

Furberg CD, Psaty BM, Meyer JV: Nifedipine: Dose-related increase in mortality in patients with coronary heart disease. *Circulation* 1995;92:1326–1331.

Gong L, Zhang W, Zhu Y, et al.: Shanghai trial of nifedipine in the elderly (STONE). *J Hypertens* 1996;14:1237–1245.

Grossman E, Messerli FH, Grodzicki T, Kowey P: Should a moratorium be placed on sublingual nifedipine capsules given for hypertensive emergencies and pseudoemergencies? *JAMA* 1996;276:1328–1331.

Kizer JR, Kimmel SE: Epidemiologic review of the calcium channel blocker drugs: An up-to-date perspective on the proposed hazards. *Arch Intern Med* 2001;161:1145–1158.

Leenen FHH, Fourney A, Notman G, Tanner J: Persistence of antihypertensive effect after missed doses of calcium antagonist with long (amlodipine) vs short (diltiazem) elimination half-life. *Br J Clin Pharmacol* 1996;41:83–88.

Lithell HOL: Effect of antihypertensive drugs on insulin, glucose, and lipid metabolism. *Diabetes Care* 1991;14:203–209.

Morgan TO, Anderson AIE, MacInnis RJ: ACE inhibitors, beta-blockers, calcium blockers, and diuretics for the control of systolic hypertension. *Am J Hypertens* 2001;14:241–247.

Packer M, O'Connor CM, Ghali JK, et al.: Effect of amlodipine on morbidity and mortality in severe chronic heart failure. *N Engl J Med* 1996;335:1107–1114.

Pedrinelli R, Dell'Omo G, Mariani M: Calcium channel blockers, postural vasoconstriction and dependent oedema in essential hypertension. *J Hum Hypertens* 2001;15:455–461.

Pitt B, Byington RP, Furberg CD, et al.: Effect of amlodipine on the progression of atherosclerosis and the occurrence of clinical events. *Circulation* 2000;102:1503–1510.

Ruzicka M, Leenen FHH: Relevance of 24-hour blood pressure profile and sympathetic activity for outcome on short-vs long-acting 1,4,-dihydropyridines. *Am J Hypertens* 1996;9: 86–94.

Staessen JA, Fagard R, Thijs L, et al.: Randomised double-blind comparison of placebo and active treatment for older patients with isolated systolic hypertension. *Lancet* 1997;350: 757–764.

Taddei S, Virdis A, Ghiadoni L, et al.: Restoration of nitric oxide availability after calcium antagonist treatment in essential hypertension. *Hypertension* 2001;37:943–948.

Wang JG, Staessen JA, Gong L, Liu L, for the Systolic Hypertension in China (Syst-China) Collaborative Group: Chinese trial on isolated systolic hypertension in the elderly. *Arch Intern Med* 1999;160:211–220.

NOTES

#22 Vasodilators: Angiotensin-Converting Enzyme Inhibitors and A-II Receptor Blockers

Multiple ACEIs and ARBs are now available (Table 22.1). As a group, these agents provide excellent antihypertensive action with few bothersome side effects. Both groups are approved for use for all degrees of hypertension and are of particular value with coexisting diabetic nephropathy or CHF or after acute MI.

ARBs provide another way to block the renin-angiotensin system. Although outcome data with these agents remain limited, they likely will prove to be equal to ACEIs in reduction of cardiovascular and renal morbidity.

Mode of Action

The conversion of the inactive prohormone angiotensin-I (A-I) to the potent vasoconstrictor A-II is accomplished mainly by an ACE available throughout the body (see Figure 22.1). ACEIs competitively inhibit the converting enzyme by attaching to its binding sites on the A-I structure, thereby blocking the synthesis of A-II so that the effects of the hormone are countered.

ARBs attach to the receptors for A-II on the blood vessels and elsewhere and thereby inhibit the effects of A-II. Since alternative pathways for the production of A-II not involving ACE may be active, ARBs might provide more complete inhibition of the renin-angiotensin system than do ACEIs. With both agents, A-II-mediated vasoconstriction is overcome and the BP falls.

Peripheral resistance and BP fall as a result of these effects. Cardiac output does not increase, possibly because of inhibition of the expected baroreceptor-mediated reflex increase in sympathetic activity as a result of the inhibition of A-II. Despite marked falls in BP, heart rate rarely rises.

The ability to reduce systemic vascular resistance without cardiac stimulation makes ACEIs particularly useful as unloading agents in the treatment of CHF, wherein high levels of A-II **22.** are usually found. Reduction of A-II within cardiac tissue may be responsible for improved myocardial remodeling after ischemic injury. Preliminary studies with ARBs suggest that they may provide similar effects.

High levels of A-II are present in the renal efferent arteriole; inhibition of A-II is the most effective means to dilate these efferent arterioles and thereby reduce intraglomerular pressure. Their renoprotective effects in diabetics are described in Sections #30 and #32.

Components of the renin-angiotensin system are present in most tissues. Part of the antihypertensive and tissue-protective effects of these agents likely come from their local effects.

ACE is the same enzyme that inactivates the vasodepressor hormone bradykinin. Inhibition of this inactivation may allow the vasodepressor effect to persist, so this effect may be involved in the antihypertensive action of ACEIs. On the other hand, high levels of bradykinin may be responsible for the cough seen with these drugs. ARBs do not increase bradykinin and do not induce cough.

Clinical Use

Once-per-day doses of longer-acting ACEIs and ARBs are being used to treat all degrees of hypertension.

Small doses of these agents should be used as initial therapies in those suspected of high renin-angiotensin forms of hypertension, since these patients may experience a precipitous first-dose hypotension when the support of BP by A-II is acutely removed. In particular, patients with bilateral RVH, wherein high levels of A-II serve to maintain renal blood flow beyond the stenoses, may experience a marked fall in BP and loss of renal function with ACEI or ARB therapy. Therefore, a serum creatinine should be repeated within three days of starting ACEI or ARB therapy in patients with extensive atherosclerosis and/or renal impairment. Whereas the BPs of the elderly and blacks respond somewhat less to ACEIs and ARBs than in younger persons and whites, their response is enhanced by addition of a diuretic. The response to an ARB and to an ACEI may differ in individual patients.

Side Effects

Side effects may be related to:
- Pharmacological effects of the drug, including:
  - Cough (not seen with ARBs)
  - Hypotension
  - Loss of renal function
- The sulfhydryl group contained within captopril but not in others, which may be responsible for more:
  - Rash
  - Loss of taste

- Glomerulopathy with proteinuria
- Leukopenia

These agents are absolutely contraindicated in pregnancy because of toxic effects on fetal development.

Angioedema is uncommon but is a serious reaction that has been reported with various ACEIs and more rarely with ARBs.

Overview

These agents are being widely used in the treatment of milder degrees of hypertension as well as the more severe, resistant forms. They work particularly well in those with higher renin levels, including those on diuretics. These agents appear to protect renal function better than other drugs that lower BP as well and are the preferred initial choice for treatment of hypertension in patients with concomitant diabetes, heart failure, or renal insufficiency. In the Heart Outcomes Prevention Evaluation (HOPE) trial, the ACEI ramipril reduced morbidity and mortality in high-risk patients while having only a minimal antihypertensive effect. In the PROGRESS trial, perindopril plus indapamide significantly reduced recurrent strokes.

Research in patients with high-to-normal renin levels suggests that these agents may correct an underlying fault of tissue responsiveness to A-II. The outlook seems particularly promising.

With more experience as to their ability to prevent or treat various complications, ARBs may be used increasingly in the place of ACEIs. As of now, their major advantages are the relative absence of side effects (particularly cough).

FIGURE 22.1

Mode of Action of Inhibitors of the Renin-Angiotensin System

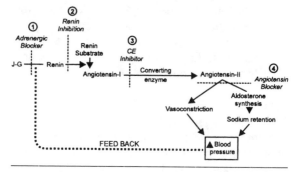

The four sites of action of currently available inhibitors of the renin-angiotensin system. (From Kaplan N.M: *Clinical Hypertension*, 8th ed. Baltimore: William & Wilkins, 2002).

TABLE 22.1

ACEIs and ARBs for Therapy of Hypertension

Drug	Trade Name	Usual Dose Range, Total mg/day (frequency per day)	Selected Side Effects and Comments
Angiotensin-converting enzyme inhibitors			
Benazepril	Lotensin	5-40 (1)	Common: cough
Captopril	Capoten	25-150 (2-3)	Rare: angioedema, hyperkalemia,
Enalapril	Vasotec	5-40 (2)	rash, loss of taste, leucopenia,
Fosinopril	Monopril	10-40 (1)	fetal toxicity
Lisinopril	Prinivil, Zestril	5-40 (1)	
Moexipril	Univasc	7.5-30 (2)	
Perindopril	Aceon	4-16 (1)	
Quinapril	Accupril	5-80 (1)	
Ramipril	Altace	1.25-20 (1)	
Trandolapril	Mavik	1-4 (1)	

Drug	Trade Name	Usual Dose Range, Total mg/day (frequency per day)	Selected Side Effects and Comments
Angiotensin II-receptor blockers			
Candesartan	Atacand	8-32 (1)	Angioedema (very rare), hyperkalemia, fetal toxicity
Eprosartan	Teveten	400-800 (1)	
Irbesartan	Avapro	150-300 (1)	
Losartan	Cozaar	50-100 (1-2)	
Olmesartan	Benecor	10-40 (1)	
Telmisartan	Micardis	40-80 (1)	
Valsartan	Diovan	80-320 (1)	

References

The ACE Inhibitors in Diabetic Nephropathy Trialist Group: Should all patients with type 1 diabetes mellitus and microalbuminuria receive angiotensin-converting enzyme inhibitors?: A meta-analysis of individual patient data. *Ann Intern Med* 2001;134:370–379.

Agodoa LY, Appel L, Bakris GL, et al.: Effect of ramipril vs amlodipine on renal outcomes in hypertensive nephrosclerosis. *JAMA* 2001;285:2719–2728.

Bakris GL: Angiotensin-converting enzyme inhibition to enhance vascular health—clinical and research models. *Am J Hypertens* 2001;14:264S–269S.

Brenner, BM, Cooper ME, de Zeeuw D, et al. Effects of losartan on renal and cardiovascular outcomes in patients with type 2 diabetes and nephropathy. *N Engl J Med* 2001;345: 861–869.

Chan P, Tomlinson B, Huant T-Y, et al.: Double-blind comparison of losartan, lisinopril, and metolazone in elderly hypertensive patients with previous angiotensin-converting enzyme inhibitor-induced cough. *J Clin Pharmacol* 1997;37:253–257.

The Heart Outcomes Prevention Evaluation Study Investigators: Effects of an angiotensin-converting enzyme inhibitor, ramipril, on cardiovascular events in high-risk patients. *N Engl J Med* 2000;342:145–153.

Jafar TH, Schmid CH, Landa M, et al.: Angiotensin-converting enzyme inhibitors and progression of nondiabetic renal disease. *Ann Intern Med* 2001;135:73–87.

Mogensen CE, Neldam S, Tikkanen I, et al., for the CALM Study Group: Randomised controlled trial of dual blockade of renin-angiotensin system in patients with hypertension, microalbuminuria, and non-insulin dependent diabetes: The Candesartan and Lisinopril Microalbuminuria (CALM) study. *BMJ* 2000;321:1440–1444.

Morgan TO, Anderson AIE, MacInnis RJ: ACE inhibitors, beta-blockers, calcium blockers, and diuretics for the control of systolic hypertension. *Am J Hypertens* 2001;14:241–247.

Pitt B, Poole-Wilson PA, Segal R, et al.: Effect of losartan compared with captopril on mortality in patients with symptomatic heart failure. *Lancet* 2000;335:1582–1587.

PROGRESS Collaborative Group. Randomised trial of a perindopril-based blood-pressure-lowering regimen among 6105 individuals with previous stroke or transient ischaemic attack. *Lancet* 2001;358:1033–1041.

Stergiou GS, Skeva II, Baibas NM, et al.: Does the antihypertensive response to angiotensin converting enzyme inhibition predict the antihypertensive response to angiotensin receptor antagonism? *Am J Hypertens* 2001;14:688–693.

Toto R: Angiotensin II subtype 1 receptor blockers and renal function. *Arch Intern Med* 2001;161:1492–1499.

Weir MR, Smith DHG, Neutel JM, Bedigian MP: Valsartan alone or with a diuretic or ACE inhibitor as treatment for African American hypertensives: Relation to salt intake. *Am J Hypertens* 2001;14:665–671.

NOTES

#23 New Agents: Vasopeptidase Inhibitors, Renin Inhibitors, Endothelin Receptor Antagonists

In the continual search for even more effective and better-tolerated antihypertensive therapy, a number of new and as-yet-not-marketed classes of drugs are under active investigation. Two of these block the renin-angiotensin system, another, the endothelin system.

Vasopeptidase Inhibitors

These agents, in a single chemical entity, block two enzymes: one, ACE, which is responsible for the breakdown of bradykinin and the conversion of inactive A-I to the major player in cardiovascular pathophysiology, A-II; the other, the neutral endopeptidase enzyme (NEP), which degrades endogenous natriuretic peptides (Figure 23.1). Thereby, the effects of an ACEI—decreases in A-II and increases in bradykinin—are combined with increases in natriuretic peptides, which are also vasodilatory. As seen in Figure 23.1, the overall physiologic effect is vasodilation.

Several such agents are currently in clinical development. The most advanced is the heterocyclic dipeptide mimetic omapatrilat, a vasopeptidase inhibitor that inhibits both ACE and NEP in a competitive fashion, having similar potency against each enzyme.

The obvious attraction of the combined ACE and NEP inhibitors is the ability to have effects on both high- and low-renin states while providing a natriuresis without activating the renin system as do traditional diuretics. Initial clinical studies in patients with hypertension have been favorable.

However, not surprisingly, the high levels of bradykinin induced by these agents (at least in the relatively high doses used in the initial trials) led to a disturbing incidence of severe angioedema, so additional trials have been done with lower doses to ensure that this problem can be minimized. Facial flushing and dyspepsia are the only other side effects that are more frequent than seen with ACEIs.

As noted by Walter and Reid: "Further clinical experience will indicate whether these side effects will occur with more or less or similar frequency compared to traditional ACE inhibitors. The crucial issue is whether vasopeptidase inhibitors, with their extended effects on vasoactive neurohumoral modulation, offer real clinical benefit over existing ACE inhibitors and angiotensin II receptor antagonists. The potential superiority of vasopeptidase inhibitors is based upon their potentiation of vasodilatory natriuretic peptides and enhanced clinical efficacy; however it remains to be seen whether this mechanistic difference will lead to clinically relevant improvement in outcome."

23.

Renin Inhibitors

Inhibitors of the action of renin to cleave the decapeptide A-I from angiotensinogen (see Figure 22.1) have been developed. These include some that must be given IV (and therefore not likely to become clinically useful) and others that are effective orally, including Ro 42-5892 (Remikiren) and A72517 (Zankiren). These agents are attractive not only because they can inhibit the production of A-I and A-II but also because they prevent the reactive rise in renin release that follows the use of ACEIs and ARBs. Whether any will become available for clinical use remains to be seen.

Endothelin Receptor Antagonists

The endothelin system comprises a family of peptides. Endothelin-I (ET-1) is the predominant one and stimulates vasoconstriction and cell proliferation by acting locally in both vascular and nonvascular cells. Endothelin ETA receptors mediate the effects of ET-1, and both extensive experimental and limited clinical studies show that endothelin receptor antagonists can block the actions of ET-1, providing vasodilation and inhibition of cellular proliferation. It will likely be a while before they become available for treatment of systemic hypertension for clinical use.

FIGURE 23.1

Neurohumoral effect of vasopeptidase inhibition

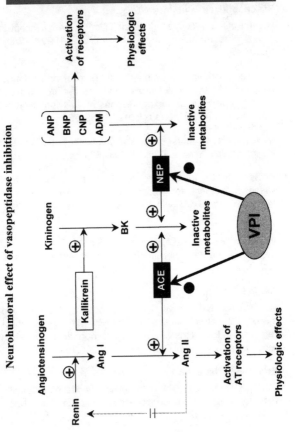

References

Vasopeptidase Inhibitors

Burnett JC Jr.: Vasopeptidase inhibition: A new concept in blood pressure management. *J Hypertens* 1999;17(Suppl 1):S37–S43.

Ferdinand K, Saini R, Lewin A, et al.: Efficacy and safety of omapatrilat with hydrochlorothiazide for the treatment of hypertension in subjects nonresponsive to hydrochlorothiazide alone. *Am J Hypertens* 2001;14:788–793.

Messerli FH, Nussberger J.: Vasopeptidase inhibition and angio-oedema. *Lancet* 2000;356:608–609.

Rouleau JL, Pfeffer MA, Stewart DJ, et al.: Comparison of vasopeptidase inhibitor, omapatrilat, and lisinopril on exercise tolerance and morbidity in patients with heart failure. *Lancet* 2000;356:615–620.

Walter M, Reid J: Vasopeptidase inhibition: Cardiovascular therapy for the new millennium? *J Hum Hypertens* 2000;14:537–539.

Renin Inhibitors

van Paassen P, de Zeeuw D, Navis G, de Jong PE: Renal and systemic effects of continued treatment with renin inhibitor remikiren in hypertensive patients with normal and impaired renal function. *Nephrol Dial Transplant* 2000;15:637–643.

Endothelin Receptor Antagonists

Barton M, Kiowski W: The therapeutic potential of endothelin receptor antagonists in cardiovascular disease. *Curr Hypertens Rep* 2001;3:322–330.

NOTES

#24 The Overall Therapeutic Plan

The various drugs available to treat hypertension have been described in the previous sections. General guidelines will be provided in subsequent sections on how individual choices of therapy are best determined. First, the various classes will be compared, both as to their relative effectiveness in reducing BP and hypertension-related morbidity and mortality and as to their likelihood of evoking significant adverse effects. Then two important pharmacological characteristics of all drugs will be considered: their dose-response relationship and their duration of action, since these, too, enter into the decision for individual choices of therapy.

Comparisons between Drugs: Efficacy

The choice of drug is often based on perceived differences in efficacy in lowering BP and the likelihood of side effects. In fact, overall anti-hypertensive efficacy varies little between the various available drugs since, to gain U.S. Food and Drug Administration approval for marketing in the United States, the drug must have been shown to be effective in reducing the BP in a large portion of the 1,500 or more patients given the drug during its clinical investigation. Moreover, the dose and formulation of drug are chosen so as not to lower the BP too much or too fast to avoid hypotensive side effects. Virtually all oral drugs are designed to do the same thing: lower the BP at least 10% in the majority of patients with mild to moderate hypertension.

Not only must each new drug be shown to be effective in large numbers of hypertensive patients but the drug also must have been tested against currently available agents to show at least equal efficacy. When comparisons between various drugs are made, they almost always come out close to one another. The best such comparison was performed in the TOMHS (Neaton et al., 1993), which involved random allocation of five drugs (chlorthalidone, acebutolol, doxazosin, amlodipine, enalapril), each given to almost 200 mild hypertensives, while another group took a placebo and all patients remained on a nutritional-hygienic program. The overall antihypertensive efficacy of the five drugs over four years was virtually equal.

Despite the fairly equal overall efficacy of various antihypertensive drugs, individual patients may vary considerably in their response to different drugs. Some of this variability can be accounted for by patient characteristics, including age and race. This was seen in a Veterans Administration (VA) cooperative one-year trial in which 1,292 men were randomly given one of six drugs from each major class. Overall and in the black patients, the CCB was most effective, but the ACEI was best in younger whites, and the beta-blocker was best in older whites (Materson et al., 1995).

Comparisons between Drugs: Reductions in Morbidity and Mortality

The critical issue is not efficacy in lowering BP but rather effectiveness in reducing morbidity and mortality. All major classes of antihypertensive drugs save alpha-blockers have been shown to reduce mortality and morbidity in large RCTs, and there are few differences between them (Blood Pressure Trialists, 2000; Psaty et al., 1997).

171

In all of the 18 RCTs completed before 1995, diuretics or beta-blockers were used (Psaty et al., 1997). In the eight RCTs completed between 1995 and 2000, ACEIs or CCBs were compared either against a diuretic ± beta-blocker or against one another (Blood Pressure Trialists, 2000). As seen in Table 24.1, one conclusion from these more recent trials seems obvious: Neither ACEI-based nor CCB-based therapies are better than diuretics ± beta-blocker-based therapies. CCB therapy did protect better against stroke and less well against CHD and CHF, but ACEIs and CCBs provided identical effects on overall morbidity and mortality.

The bottom line of Table 24.1 shows data from the two trials directly comparing an ACEI to a CCB, one the ABCD trial (Schrier and Estacio, 2000) that had 470 patients, the other the STOP-2 (Hansson et al., 1999) that had 4,401 taking either an ACEI or a CCB. Obviously, most of the results are derived from the STOP-2 trial. Although there is apparently lesser protection against CHD and CHF with the CCB than with the ACEI, the words of the principal investigators of STOP-2 should be heeded: "Our results should be interpreted with some caution, since 48 statistical comparisons were done. Calcium antagonists were not, however, less effective in any other way in the prevention of cardiovascular events than conventional drugs or ACEIs, which accords with current opinion about safety of calcium antagonists when used appropriately." (Hansson et al., 1999)

The results of the eight comparative trials completed since 1995 are by no means definitive. Fortunately, a large number of trials are in progress, so that before long we should have more definitive data to guide our choices in therapy. These data will include outcome studies with ARBs.

Of course, the playing field keeps growing. By the time we know if ARBs are as good as ACEIs, vasopeptidase inhibitors will likely be available, so the process of finding out what's best will likely never end.

In one sense, the process is irrelevant. As the need to achieve lower goals of therapy has become obvious, the need to use more than one drug in the majority of hypertensives has also become obvious. This is nowhere better seen than among diabetic hypertensives who will be considered in a subsequent section. Therefore, the best combination of agents, almost always to include a low dose of diuretic, will be a more pertinent object of trials in the future.

Comparisons between Drugs: Adverse Effects

Two points are obvious concerning differences in adverse effects among different agents. First, no drug that causes dangerous adverse effects beyond a rare idiosyncratic reaction when given in usual doses will remain on the market, even if it slips by the approval process, as witnessed by the CCB mibefradil. Second, drugs that cause frequent bothersome though not dangerous adverse effects, such as guanethidine, will likely no longer be used now that so many other choices are available.

The various antihypertensive agents vary significantly, both in the frequency of adverse effects and, to an even greater degree, in their nature. The only currently available comparisons of a representative drug from all major classes given as monotherapy to sizable numbers of patients are the previously described TOMHS and VA Cooperative Study. Side effects differed between the drugs, but no one drug was markedly more or less acceptable than the others. The differences may include sexual dysfunction. Impotence was twice as common in men in the TOMH study given the diuretic chlorthalidone than those given a placebo, whereas less impotence was seen among those given the alpha-blocker doxazosin (Grimm et al., 1997).

Over the past 25 years, a number of studies have examined the side effects of antihypertensive agents on the QOL using various questionnaires and scales. The results confirm the general impression: although 10% to 20% of patients will experience bothersome adverse effects from virtually any and every antihypertensive drug, the overall impact of therapies on QOL over two to six months of observation is positive. However, different drugs do have different profiles of side effects, and only by careful observations can subtle differences be detected, as with sexual dysfunction in the TOMHS trial.

Not infrequently, anxiety-related symptoms such as fatigue, headache, and tachycardia are mistakenly blamed on drugs. Anxiety-induced hyperventilation is common in hypertensives whose BP is difficult to control, often exacerbated by the belief that "the silent killer" is soon to strike again. Here again, starting therapy with very small doses of, hopefully, a new drug that has never been taken before along with behavioral cognitive therapy to relieve the anxiety (and often rebreathing into a paper sack to overcome acute symptoms) may help these difficult patients.

More Serious Adverse Effects

In addition to these QOL issues, more serious problems have been blamed on various classes of antihypertensive drugs. Virtually all of these claims have come from noncontrolled, often retrospective, observational case-control studies, and most of them have been subsequently proven wrong.

Cancer from Reserpine and CCBs. The first and perhaps most egregious claim was that the use of reserpine was associated with a twofold to fourfold increased risk of breast cancer in women, a claim made in three simultaneously published papers from outstanding investigators. As subsequently shown by Feinstein (1988), these studies were all contaminated by the bias of excluding women at high risk for cancer from the control groups. Multiple subsequently published perspective studies showed no association.

More recently, Pahor et al. reported a twofold greater risk for cancer in elderly patients taking short-acting CCBs compared to users of beta-blockers. Unfortunately, no ascertainment of drug use after the original observation that the subjects had the respective drugs in their possession was made, so that the actual intake of drugs is totally unknown. Multiple subsequent reports of much larger populations in which drug use was appropriately ascertained have found *no increase* in cancer among users of CCBs (Kizer and Kimmel, 2001).

Coronary Disease from CCBs. Psaty et al. (1995) reported a 60% increase in the risk of acute

MI among patients taking short-acting CCBs and strongly suggested that their claims against short-acting CCBs also carried over to the longer-acting agents. There are significant differences in the hemodynamic and hormonal responses to short-acting versus long-acting CCBs, so that the faults of the former should not be assumed to apply to the latter.

On the other hand, some cohort observational studies have shown a higher mortality rate among CCB users than other drugs. As Michels et al. (1998) conclude: "Whether the observed elevated risk [in CCB users] is real, or a result of residual confounding by indication, or chance, or a combination of the above cannot be evaluated with certainty on the basis of these observational data." The probability that confounding was a major factor in these associations is supported by the finding that, among 77,000 patients, the likelihood of being prescribed a CCB rather than other antihypertensives was significantly higher for patients with coexisting coronary disease (7.8-fold) or diabetes (1.5-fold) (Leader et al., 2001).

As seen in Table 24.1, in the comparative trials in which all patients were treated with active drugs, the increase in coronary events seen with CCBs compared to other drugs was largely balanced by a lower risk of strokes in the CCB-treated patients with no differences in mortality between different classes. As previously noted, data from ongoing large comparative trials will settle the issue once and for all.

Dose-Response Relationship

Beyond the individual variabilities in response to drugs, there is a more generalized problem with the use of antihypertensive agents: They often are prescribed in doses that are too high. The problem of overdosing has been obvious with virtually every new drug introduced, wherein the initial recommended doses have been gradually reduced because, after widespread clinical experience, they proved to be too high. For example, whereas 100 to 200 mg of HCT were initially used, 12.5 mg is now recognized as enough for many patients.

The obvious solution to this problem is for practitioners to start patients with doses that will not be fully effective and to gradually titrate the dose to the desired response.

Need for 24-Hour Coverage

As noted in Section #1, self-recorded measurements and ambulatory automatic BP monitoring are being increasingly used to ensure the 24-hour duration of action of anti-hypertensive agents. This is particularly critical with the increasing use of once-a-day medications that often do not provide 24-hour efficacy, such as enalapril and atenolol. Therefore, the patient is exposed to the full impact of the early morning abrupt rise in BP that is almost certainly involved in the increased incidence of various cardiovascular events immediately after arising.

Drugs that continue to work beyond 24 hours are even more attractive to prevent loss of control in the considerable number who skip a dose at least once weekly, as has been documented in 30% or more of patients with hypertension. A small but hopefully increasing number of drugs are available that will maintain good efficacy on a missed day, including the CCB amlodipine and the ACEIs perindopril and trandolapril.

TABLE 24.1

Prospective Overview of Comparative Randomized Trials for Hypertension[a]

	Relative Risks (Confidence Interval)					
	Stroke	CHD	CHF	Major CV Events	CV Death	Total Mortality
ACEI vs D/βB[b] (3 trials; 16,161 pts)	1.05 (.92-1.19)	1.00 (.88-1.14)	.92 (.77-1.09)	1.00 (.93-1.08)	1.00 (.87-1.15)	1.03 (.93-1.14)
CCB vs D/βB (5 trials; 23,454 pts)	.87 (.77-.98)	1.12 (1.0-1.26)	1.12 (.95-1.33)	1.02 (.95-1.10)	1.05 (.92-1.2)	1.01 (.92-1.11)
ACEI vs CCB (2 trials; 4,871 pts)	1.02 (.85-1.21)	.81 (.68-.97)	.82 (.67-1.0)	.92 (.83-1.01)	1.04 (.87-1.24)	1.03 (.91-1.18)

[a] Modified from the Blood Pressure Lowering Trialists' Collaboration. Lancet 2000;356:1955-1064.

[b] ACEI, angiotensin-converting-enzyme inhibitor; βB, beta-blocker; CCB, calcium channel blocker; D, diuretic.

References

Blood Pressure Lowering Treatment Trialists' Collaboration. Effects of ACE inhibitors, calcium antagonists, and other blood-pressure-lowering drugs. *Lancet* 2000;355:1955–1964.

Feinstein AR: Scientific standards in epidemiologic studies of the menace of daily life. *Science* 1988;242:1257–1263.

Grimm RH Jr., Grandits GA, Prineas RJ, et al.: Long-term effects on sexual function of five antihypertensive drugs and nutritional hygienic treatment of hypertensive men and women. *Hypertension* 1997;29:8–14.

Hansson L, Lindholm LH, Ekbom T, et al.: Randomised trial of old and new antihypertensive drugs in elderly patients. *Lancet* 1999;354:1751–1756.

Joint National Committee on Detection, Evaluation, and Treatment of High Blood Pressure. The sixth report of the Joint National Committee on Detection, Evaluation, and Treatment of High Blood Pressure (JNC VI). *Arch Intern Med* 1997;116:686–690.

Kaplan NM: The appropriate goals of antihypertensive therapy. *Ann Intern Med* 1992;116:686–690.

Kizer JR, Kimmel SE: Epidemiologic review of the calcium channel blocker drugs: An up-to-date perspective on the proposed hazards. *Arch Intern Med* 2001;161:1145–1158.

Leader S, Mallick R, Roht L: Using medication history to measure confounding by indication in assessing calcium channel blockers and other antihypertensive therapy. *J Hum Hypertens* 2001;15:153–159.

Materson BJ, Reda DJ, Cushman WC, et al.: Department of Veterans Affairs single-drug therapy of hypertension study. *Am J Hypertens* 1995;8:189–192.

Michels KB, Rosner BA, Manson JE, et al.: Prospective study of calcium channel blocker use, cardiovascular disease, and total mortality among hypertensive women. *Circulation* 1998;97:1540–1548.

Neaton JD, Grimm RH Jr., Prineas RJ, et al.: Treatment of mild hypertension study (TOMHS): Final results. *JAMA* 1993;270: 713–724.

Pahor M, Guralnik JM, Ferrucci L, et al.: Calcium-channel blockade and incidence of cancer in aged populations. *Lancet* 1996;348:493–497.

Psaty BM, Heckbert SR, Koepsell TD, et al.: The risk of myocardial infarction associated with antihypertensive drug therapies. *JAMA* 1995;274:620–625.

Psaty BM, Smith NL, Siscovick DS, et al.: Health outcomes associated with antihypertensive therapies used as first-line agents. *JAMA* 1997;277:739–745.

Schrier RW, Estacio RO: Additional follow-up from the ABCD trial in patients with type 2 diabetes and hypertension. *N Engl J Med* 2000;343:1969.

#25 The Choice of First Drug

A large number of drugs can be chosen for initial therapy, and the choice should be made carefully. If patients respond well, the drug may be taken for many years; therefore, inapparent biochemical and other side effects must be avoided. If patients do not respond well or have significant side effects with the first drug, they may be dissuaded from returning for follow-up care.

The majority of patients have mild hypertension that should be adequately managed with one drug. In most therapeutic trials involving patients with DBPs from 90 to 100 mm Hg, 40 to 60 percent had pressures brought to below 90 mm Hg (and often had at least a 10 mm Hg absolute fall) with one drug. Therefore, the choice of the first drug is an important one.

JNC-6 Recommendations

Taking cognizance of the fact that the initial large RCTs that have shown an overall decrease in cardiovascular morbidity and mortality involved the use of diuretics or, to a lesser extent, beta-blockers, JNC-6 recommended that therapy be started with one of these agents in patients with no specific indication for another class of drug (see Figure 25.1).

However, the majority of hypertensives have one or more concomitant conditions, so the choice should be individualized. This same approach is recommended in all current guidelines from expert committees.

Individualized Therapy

Rather than using a set formula for all patients, various features of each patient should be considered in making the most appropriate choice of first drug, one that will more likely lower BP to desired levels, improve concomitant conditions, and leave patients unencumbered by bothersome side effects. The two major features that should prove most helpful are demographics and concomitant diseases (see Table 25.1).

Some advocate that therapy be based on various biochemical measurements, such as PRA or hemodynamic functions. The author does not believe these are needed. Although the cost of therapy ought not to enter into the decision, those who cannot afford more expensive drugs may have to take less expensive ones even if they are not the preferred choices. Fortunately, with the increasing availability of once-per-day formulations, fewer tablets should be needed so that the daily cost of therapy should be kept affordable.

25.

The alpha-beta-blocker labetalol is not included in Table 25.1 because it is used mainly for more severe hypertension in combination with other drugs. On the other hand, the combinations of a low dose of the beta-blocker bisoprolol or the ACEI benazepril with HCT have been approved for initial therapy. A number of other combination tablets, some including ACEIs and CCBs, are also available for those who require additional therapy (see Table 25.2).

Other factors may be involved, in addition to the coexisting conditions shown in Table 25.1. Examples include:

- Poorly compliant patients, who should: Avoid central alpha-agonists (danger of rebound) Use only long-acting, once-per-day formulations
- Patients with depression, who should avoid reserpine and central alpha-agonists

- Patients who are physically active, who may be slowed by beta-blockers
- Patients with migraine, who should use nonselective beta-blockers or CCBs
- Patients with collagen diseases, who should avoid methyldopa and hydralazine

Obviously, the list is almost endless, since there are so many antihypertensive agents and even more concomitant conditions that may be affected by their use. Fortunately, knowledge about the known effects, both good and bad, of the different classes of drugs will usually be adequate to enable clinicians to match their patients' overall status to the most preferred choices. The ideal is a choice that will not only control the hypertension but also improve coexisting conditions.

Conclusion

In clinical practice, a low dose of a thiazide diuretic (logically with a potassium-sparing agent) is the most appropriate choice for initial therapy of almost all patients. For most, another drug will be needed to reduce BP to the lower goals that are now recommended; however, the presence of a diuretic will enhance the efficacy of whatever else is needed.

FIGURE 25.1

JNC-6 Therapeutic Algorithm

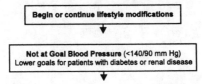

Begin or continue lifestyle modifications

↓

Not at Goal Blood Pressure (<140/90 mm Hg)
Lower goals for patients with diabetes or renal disease

↓

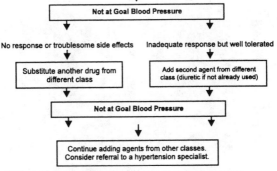

Initial Drug Choices*

Uncomplicated Hypertension†
Diuretics
Beta-blockers

Specific indications for the following drugs (see Table 9)
ACE inhibitors
Angiotensin-II receptor blockers
Alpha-blockers
Alpha-Beta-blockers
Beta-blockers
Calcium antagonists
Diuretics

Compelling Indications†
Diabetes mellitus with proteinuria
• ACE inhibitors
Heart failure
• ACE inhibitors
• Diuretics
Isolated systolic hypertension (older persons)
• Diuretics preferred
• Long-acting dihydropyridine calcium antagonists
Myocardial infarction
• Beta-blockers (non-ISA)
• ACE inhibitors (with systolic dysfunction)

• Start with a low dose of a long-acting once-daily drug, and titrate dose.
• Low-dose combinations may be appropriate.

↓

Not at Goal Blood Pressure

No response or troublesome side effects

Substitute another drug from different class

Inadequate response but well tolerated

Add second agent from different class (diuretic if not already used)

↓

Not at Goal Blood Pressure

↓

Continue adding agents from other classes.
Consider referral to a hypertension specialist.

* Unless contraindicated. ACE indicates angiotensin-converting enzyme; ISA, intrinsic sympathomimetic activity.
† Based on randomized controlled trials.

Simplified algorithm for treatment of hypertension. (From the sixth report of the Joint National Committee on Detection, Evaluation, and Treatment of High Blood Pressure (JNC-VI. Arch Intern Med 1997;157:2413-2446.

TABLE 25.1

Considerations for Individualizing Antihypertensive Drug Therapy[a]

May Have Favorable Effects on Comorbid Conditions		May Have Unfavorable Effects on Comorbid Conditions[b]	
Condition	Drug	Condition	Drug
Angina	Beta-blockers, CCB	Bronchospasmic diseases	Beta-blockers[c]
Atrial tachycardia and fibrillation	Beta-blockers	2° or 3° heart block	Beta-blockers[c], CCB (non-DHP)[c]
Cough from ACE inhibitor	ARB	Depression	Central alpha-agonists, Reserpine[c]
Cyclosporine-induced hypertension	CCB	Dyslipidemia	Beta-blockers (non-ISA), Diuretics (high-dose)
Diabetes mellitus, particularly with proteinuria	ACEI, ARB, diuretics, CCBs, Beta-blockers	Gout	Diuretics
		Heart failure	CCB[b]
Dyslipidemia	Alpha-blockers	Hyperkalemia	ACEI, ARB
Essential tremor	Beta-blockers (non-CS)	Liver disease	Labetalol, Methyldopa[c]

Condition	Drug	Condition	Drug
Heart failure	ACEIs, Carvedilol, beta-blockers, diuretics	Peripheral vascular disease	Beta-blockers
Hyperthyroidism	Beta-blockers	Pregnancy	ACEI[c], ARB[c]
Migraine	Beta-blockers (non-CS) CCB	Renal insufficiency	Potassium-sparing agents
Osteoporosis	Thiazides	Renovascular disease, bilateral	ACEI ARB
Preoperative hypertension	Beta-blockers	Type 1 and 2 diabetes	Beta-blockers
Prostatism	Alpha-blockers		High-dose diuretics
Renal insufficiency	ACEI		
Systolic hypertension in elderly	Diuretics, CCB		

a Modified from the sixth report of the Joint National Committee. Arch Intern Med 1997;157:2413-2446.
b These drugs may be used with special monitoring, unless contraindicated.
c Contraindicated
ACEI, angiotensin-converting enzyme inhibitor; ARB, angiotensin II receptor blocker; CCB, calcium channel blocker; DHP, dihydropyridine; non-CS, non-cardioselective; non-ISA, non-intrinsic sympathomimetic activity.

TABLE 25.2

Combination Drugs for Hypertension

Drug	Trade Name
Beta-Adrenergic Blockers and Diuretics	
Atenolol 50 or 100 mg/chlorthalidone 25 mg	Tenoretic
Bisoprolol 2.5, 5, or 10 mg/hydrochlorothiazide 6.25 mg	Ziac*
Metoprolol 50 or 100 mg/hydrochlorothiazide 25 or 50 mg	Lopressor HCT
Nadolol 40 or 80 mg/bendroflumethiazide 5 mg	Corzide
Propranolol 40 or 80 mg/hydrochlorothiazide 25 mg	Inderide
Propranolol (extended release) 80, 120, or 160 mg/hydrochlorothiazide 50 mg	Inderide LA
Timolol 10 mg/hydrochlorothiazide 25 mg	Timolide
ACE Inhibitors and Diuretics	
Benazepril 5, 10, or 20 mg/hydrochlorothiazide 6.25, 12.5 or 25 mg	Lotensin HCT
Captopril 25 or 50 mg/hydrochlorothiazide 15 or 25 mg	Capozide*
Enalapril 5 or 10 mg/hydrochlorothiazide 12.5 or 25 mg	Vaseretic
Lisinopril 10 or 20 mg/hydrochlorothiazide 12.5 or 25 mg	Prinzide; Zestoretic

Angiotensin-II Receptor Antagonists and Diuretics

Losartan 50 mg/hydrochlorothiazide 12.5 mg — Hyzaar

Calcium-Channel Antagonists and ACE Inhibitors

Amlodipine 2.5 or 5 mg/benazepril 10 or 20 mg — Lotrel

Diltiazem 10 mg/enalapril 5 mg — Teczem

Verapamil (extended release) 180 or 240 mg/trandolapril 1, 2, or 4 mg — Tarka

Felodipine 5 mg/enalapril 5 mg — Lexxel

Other Combinations

Triamterene 37.5, 50, or 75 mg/hydrochlorothiazide 25 or 50 mg — Dyazide, Maxide

Spironolactone 25 or 50 mg/hydrochlorothiazide 25 or 50 mg — Aldactazide

Amiloride 5 mg/hydrochlorothiazide 50 mg — Moduretic

Guanethidine 10 mg/hydrochlorothiazide 25 mg — Esimil

Hydralazine 25, 50, or 100 mg/hydrochlorothiazide 25 or 30 mg — Apresazide

Methyldopa 250 or 500 mg/hydrochlorothiazide 15, 25, 30, or 50 mg — Alodril

Reserpine 0.125 mg/hydrochlorothiazide 25 or 50 mg — Hydropres

Reserpine 0.1 mg/hydralazine 25 mg/hydrochlorothiazide 15 mg — Ser-ap-es

Drug	Trade Name
Clonidine 0.1, 0.2, or 0.3 mg/chlorthalidone 15 mg	Combipres
Methyldopa 250 mg/chlorothiazide 150 or 250 mg	Aldochlor
Reserpine 0.125 or 0.25 mg/chlorthalidone 25 or 50 mg	Demi-Regroton
Reserpine 0.125 or 0.25 mg/chlorothiazide 250 or 500 mg	Diupres
Prazosin 1, 2, or 5 mg/ polythiazide 0.5 mg	Minizide

Approved for initial therapy

References

Abernathy DR: Pharmacological properties of combination therapies for hypertension. *Am J Hypertens* 1997;10:13S–16S.

Brunner HR, Menard J, Waeber B, et al.: Treating the individual hypertensive patient: Considerations on dose, sequential monotherapy, and drug combinations. *J Hypertens* 1990; 8:3–11.

Joint National Committee. The Sixth Report of the Joint National Committee on Detection, Evaluation, and Treatment of High Blood Pressure (JNC VI). *Arch Intern Med* 1997;157: 2413–2446.

Kaplan NM, Gifford RW: Choice of initial therapy for hypertension. *JAMA* 1996;275:1577–1580.

Materson BJ, Reda DJ, Cushman WC, et al.: Single-drug therapy for hypertension in men: A comparison of six antihypertensive agents with placebo. *N Engl J Med* 1993;328: 914–921.

Neaton JD, Grimm RH Jr., Prineas RJ, et al.: Treatment of mild hypertension study (TOMHS): Final results. *JAMA* 1993;2;70: 713–724.

Psaty BM, Smith NL, Siscovick DS, et al.: Health outcomes associated with antihypertensive therapies used as first-line agents. *JAMA* 1997;277:739–745.

#26 The Choice of Second and Third Drug

Diuretic as Second Choice

Whatever agent other than a diuretic is chosen as first drug, a low dose of diuretic should almost always be chosen as second. This addition will increase the antihypertensive efficacy of other drugs. This reflects not only on the expected antihypertensive effect derived from the action of the diuretic but also the ability of the diuretic to remove excess fluid that may have been retained by the kidneys when BP is reduced. In addition to overcoming this "side effect" of nondiuretic therapy, the combination may blunt some of the side effects of the diuretic.

In particular, if the initial choice has been a beta-blocker, an ACEI, or an ARB, the potassium wastage often induced by the diuretic may be prevented, because these drugs block the diuretic-induced rises in renin-aldosterone.

Patients Who Need Two Drugs Initially

JNC-6 (1997) notes that modifications in the usual approach of starting with one drug may be needed for those at higher risk of a coronary event or stroke because of other risk factors or target-organ damage:

"Although some patients may respond adequately to a single drug, it is often necessary to add a second or third agent after a short interval if control is not achieved. The intervals between changes in the regimen should be decreased, and the maximum dose of some drugs may be increased. In some patients, it may be necessary to start treatment with more than one agent.

Patients with average diastolic blood pressure of 120 mm Hg or greater and systolic blood pressure of 200 mm Hg or greater require more immediate therapy."

Combination Therapy

If a moderate dose of the first choice is well tolerated and effective but not enough to bring the BP down to the desired level, a second drug can be added, and thereby better control will likely be achieved than by increasing the dose of the first drug.

As noted by the JNC (1997):

> "Combinations of low doses of two agents from different classes have been shown to provide additional antihypertensive efficacy, thereby minimizing the likelihood of dose-dependent side effects. Very low doses of a diuretic (e.g., 6.25 mg hydrochlorothiazide) can potentiate the effect of the other agent without producing adverse metabolic effects (Frishman et al., 1994). Low-dose combinations with an ACEI and a nondihydropyridine calcium antagonist may reduce proteinuria more than either drug alone (Epstein and Bakris, 1996). Combinations of a dihydropyridine calcium antagonist and an ACEI induce less pedal edema than does the calcium antagonist alone (Gradman et al., 1997). In some instances, drugs with similar modes of action may provide additive effects, such as metolazone and a loop diuretic in renal failure."

26.

Choice of Third Drug

Various combinations usually work. In a parallel study, captopril, nifedipine, and hydralazine were equally effective when added to a diuretic and a beta-blocker, but the ACEI was better tolerated (Bevan et al., 1993). The key, as with two drugs, is to combine agents with different mechanisms of action.

Few patients should need more than three drugs, particularly if the various reasons for resistance to therapy that are covered in Section #28 are considered. For those who do, the JNC-6 report recommends considering referral to a hypertension specialist. The American Society of Hypertension has certified almost 1,000 U.S. physicians as hypertension specialists. The list is available on their website http://www.ash-us.org.

References

Abernethy DR: Pharmacological properties of combination therapies for hypertension. *Am J Hypertens* 1997;10:13S–16S.

Bevan EG, Pringle SD, Waller PC, et al.: Comparison of captopril, hydralazine, and nifedipine as third drug in hypertensive patients. *J Hum Hypertens* 1993;7:83–88.

Cappuccio FP, Markandu ND, Singer DRJ, MacGregor GA: Amlodipine and lisinopril in combination for the treatment of essential hypertension: Efficacy and predictors of response. *J Hypertens* 1993;11:839–847.

Epstein M, Bakris G. Newer approaches to antihypertensive therapy: Use of fixed-dose combination therapy. *Arch Intern Med* 1996;156:1969–1978.

Frishman WH, Bryzinski BS, Coulson LR, et al. A multifactorial trial design to assess combination therapy in hypertension: Treatment with bisoprolol and hydrochlorothiazide. *Arch Intern Med* 1994;154:1461–1468.

Gradman AH, Cutler NR, Davis PJ, et al.: Combined enalapril and felodipine extended release (ER) for systemic hypertension. *Am J Cardiol* 1997;79:431–435.

Joint National Committee on Detection, Evaluation, and Treatment of High Blood Pressure: The 1997 report of the Sixth Joint National Committee on Detection, Evaluation, and Treatment of High Blood Pressure. *Arch Intern Med* 1997;157:2413–2446.

Spitalewitz S, Porush JG, Reiser IW: Minoxidil, nadolol, and a diuretic: Once-a-day therapy for resistant hypertension. *Arch Intern Med* 1986;146:882–886.

#27 Step-Down Therapy/The Problem of Impotence

Step-Down Therapy
Impotence

STEP-DOWN THERAPY

Once a good response has occurred and has been maintained for a year or longer, medications may be reduced or discontinued. In a review of all published series of planned withdrawal, 42% of selected patients with mild hypertension were found to remain normotensive for 12 months or longer off medication (Nelson et al., 2001). The characteristics that make withdrawal more likely to be successful were: lower levels of BP before and after therapy; fewer and lower doses of medication needed to control hypertension; and willingness to follow lifestyle modifications.

One of the trials included in this review was the Trial of Nonpharmacologic Interventions in the Elderly (TONE), in which 886 elderly patients with BP below 145/85 on one medication went through a two-step attempt at withdrawal of their therapy (Kostis et al., 1998). In the 774 who were successfully withdrawn, the BP remained below 150/90 in almost half of those who followed a regimen of weight loss and lower sodium intake over the next 36 months. Only 16% of those who simply stopped their medication without lifestyle modifications remained below 150/90. No increase in cardiovascular events was seen among those who were able to withdraw from medication and remained normotensive.

Whether it is worth the trouble to stop successful drug therapy completely is questionable. The more sensible approach in well-controlled patients would be to first decrease the dose of whatever is being used. If this succeeds, withdrawal may be attempted with continued surveillance of the BP.

IMPOTENCE

Of various side effects of therapy, inability to gain and maintain an erection is perhaps the least well understood and managed. Loss of erectile potency may accompany the use of any antihypertensive agent. In the first two years of the MRC trial, impotence was noted in 10 percent of men on placebo, 13 percent on a beta-blocker, and 23 percent on a thiazide diuretic. In the TOMHS, impotence was noted in 17.1 percent of men on chlorthalidone vs. 8.1 percent of those on placebo. The incidence was lower than placebo only in those on the alpha-blocker doxazosin (Grimm et al, 1997).

27.

There is no known reason for this surprisingly higher frequency with diuretic therapy. Erectile dysfunction can occur with any drug that lowers BP quickly and markedly. Hypertensive men may have considerable atherosclerotic narrowing of the arteries bringing blood into the penis. Penile blood flow may diminish further if the head of pressure within this area of the circulation is reduced significantly by effective antihypertensive therapy. Since erection requires a tenfold increase in blood flow, the occurrence of impotence can be looked upon as a nonspecific effect of successful lowering of BP.

Causes

Impotence may be purely psychogenic, reflecting the concerns of middle-aged men who suddenly find themselves to have hypertension, but some become impotent because their BPs are brought down too much and too fast. Therefore, the lowering of BP should be gradual and gentle.

If impotence appears with any one drug, patients should discontinue use of that drug and be watched to see if potency returns. If it does, another type of drug should be used. An immediate switch of therapy can be made if the pressure is so high as not to allow discontinuance of therapy; these patients should be encouraged that a switch to another drug may make a difference.

Fortunately, effective therapies for erectile dysfunction are now available. In particular, sildenafil (Viagra®) is an effective treatment for most patients. Although its actions are primarily within penile smooth muscle, some systemic vasodilatory effects may induce flushing and headache. Although the coadministration of nitrates may lead to profound hypotension, little interference with antihypertensive drugs has been seen in 10 double-blind, placebo-controlled studies reviewed by Kloner et al. (2001).

Loss of sexual desire or libido is rarely caused by antihypertensive medications and is more likely psychogenic in origin. Spironolactone can interfere with testosterone synthesis and cause loss of libido.

Among the women in the TOMHS, 4.9 percent reported sexual dysfunction before therapy; the incidence of new sexual problems was low and similar to those seen with all types of antihypertensive drugs.

References

Christensen KL, Mulvany MJ: Vasodilatation, not hypotension, improves resistance vessel design during treatment of essential hypertension: A literature survey. *J Hypertens* 2001;19: 1001–1006.

Grimm RH, Grandits GA, Prineas RJ, et al.: Long-term effects on sexual function of five antihypertensive drugs and nutritional hygienic treatment in hypertensive men and women. *Hypertension* 1997;29:8–14.

Kloner RA, Brown M, Prisant LM, Collins M, for the Sildenafil Study Group: Effect of sildenafil in patients with erectile dysfunction taking antihypertensive therapy. *Am J Hypertens* 2001;14:70–73.

Kostis JB, Espeland MA, Appel L, et al.: Does withdrawal of antihypertensive medication increase the risk of cardiovascular events? *Am J Cardiol* 1998;82:1501–1508.

Nelson M, Reid C, Krum H, McNeil J: A systematic review of predictors of maintenance of normotension after withdrawal of antihypertensive drugs. *Am J Hypertens* 2001;14:98–105.

Virag R, Bouilly P, Frydman D: Is impotence an arterial disorder? *Lancet* 1985;1:181–184.

#28 Special Patients:
Resistant Hypertension

Before patients are labeled as resistant (i.e., DBPs above 95 mm Hg despite appropriate use of three or more drugs), BPs should be checked out of the office. As many as half of patients with apparent resistance based on office readings have been found to be responsive based on home or ambulatory recordings.

The multiple causes of true resistance are listed in Table 28.1.

Volume Overload

Some patients may not respond to appropriate antihypertensive therapy because of reactive fluid retention. Of the multiple reasons for resistance to therapy, volume overload due to either inadequate diuretic therapy or excessive sodium intake is the most common.

The problem may not become obvious until BP is partially lowered. This creates an even greater tendency for sodium retention by the hypertensive patient's kidneys, which have been reset to tolerate a higher head of pressure without excreting extra volume. When the pressure is lowered, even to levels well within the normal range, hypertensive patients' kidneys may respond by retaining more sodium and water in a misguided attempt to bring BPs back to the higher levels to which they have adjusted.

Therefore, BPs that have been successfully lowered may begin gradually to increase, a process called pseudotolerance, since it is caused by reactive fluid retention and not by a true tolerance or tachyphylaxis to antihypertensive therapy. Doses of diuretics that were adequate may need to be increased. Amounts of dietary sodium that did not appear to be excessive may need to be reduced.

The problem is most common with those antihypertensive agents that stimulate the renin-aldosterone mechanism, such as direct-acting vasodilators (hydralazine or minoxidil) and less common with those that suppress it, such as beta-blockers and ACEIs. CCBs may actually be natriuretic and therefore less likely to cause fluid retention.

Inadequate Dosages or Drug Interference

In addition to the need for supplementary or more potent diuretics, the doses of other antihypertensive agents may need to be increased either because inadequate amounts have been prescribed or because their effects are being antagonized. The doses may be too low because some patients inactivate the drugs more rapidly. The acetylation of hydralazine is genetically determined to be slow or rapid; hepatic blood flow and metabolism may be increased by other drugs, food, or nicotine.

28.

A number of other drugs may antagonize the effects of antihypertensive agents. Some of these do so by stimulating the sympathetic nervous system, e.g., phenylpropanolamine in diet pills and nasal decongestants, amphetamine, and cocaine. Others, such as antidepressants, block the action of drugs that work via neuronal uptake, e.g., guanethidine and methyldopa. NSAIDs decrease the effects of diuretics, beta-blockers, and ACEIs likely by decreasing levels of vasodilatory prostaglandins.

Associated Conditions

Other conditions that may elevate BP may either have been present all along and missed or have developed after therapy was begun. The importance of the pressor effect of alcohol intake greater than two ounces per day is described in Section #9. Renal damage from progressive nephrosclerosis is particularly common in blacks, whereas diabetics are susceptible to progressive glomerular sclerosis. As renal function deteriorates, hypertension often worsens, likely from sodium retention.

Renovascular Hypertension

Of all the secondary forms of hypertension, renovascular disease is the most common among those with resistant hypertension. As noted in Section #5, this is particularly common among those with rapidly progressive disease and was found in one-third of a series of 123 patients with accelerated or malignant hypertension.

Overview

The cause of resistant hypertension should be recognizable. It may take hospitalization, but that step should only rarely be necessary and, in fact, may be misleading. BPs almost always fall during hospital stays but may rise again after discharge, even without obvious changes in therapy.

If the cause can be identified, relief may be simple. If not, larger doses of more potent drugs may be required. If that fails, referral to a Hypertension Specialist is appropriate.

TABLE 28.1

Causes for Inadequate Responsiveness to Therapy

Pseudoresistance
  White-coat or office elevations

  Pseudohypertension in the elderly

Nonadherence to therapy
  Side effects of medication

  Costs of medication

  Lack of consistent and continuous primary care

  Inconvenient and/or chaotic dosing schedules

  Instructions not understood

  Organic brain syndrome (e.g., memory deficit)

Drug-related causes
  Doses too low or duration of action too short

  Inappropriate combinations (e.g., two centrally acting adrenergic inhibitors)

  Rapid inactivation (e.g., hydralazine)

  Drug interactions (e.g., NSAIDs, sympathomimetics, cyclosporine)

  Excessive volume contraction with stimulation of renin-aldosterone

  Hypokalemia (usually diuretic-induced)

  Rebound after clonidine withdrawal

Associated conditions
  Smoking

  Increasing obesity, particularly with sleep apnea

  Insulin resistance/hyperinsulinemia

  Ethanol intake of more than one ounce per day (more than two portions)

  Anxiety-induced hyperventilation or panic attacks

  Chronic pain

  Intense vasoconstriction (Raynaud's arteritis)

continued TABLE 28.1

Secondary hypertension, in particular
  Renal insufficiency

  Renovascular hypertension

Volume overload
  Excess sodium intake

  Progressive renal damage (nephrosclerosis)

  Fluid retention from reduction of blood pressure

  Inadequate diuretic therapy

References

Conlin PR, Moore TJ, Swartz SL, et al.: Effect of indomethacin on blood pressure lowering by captopril and losartan in hypertensive patients. *Hypertension* 2000;36:461–465.

Graves JW: Management of difficult to control hypertension. *Mayo Clin Proc* 2000;75:278–284.

Hyman DJ, Pavlik VN: Characteristics of patients with uncontrolled hypertension in the United States. *N Engl J Med* 2001; 345:479–486.

Isaksson H, Cederholm T, Jansson E, Nygren A, Ostergren J: Therapy-resistant hypertension associated with central obesity, insulin resistance, and large muscle fibre area. *Blood Press* 1993;2:46–52.

Mejia AD, Egan BM, Schork NJ, Zweifler AJ: Artifacts in measurement of blood pressure and lack of target organ involvement in the assessment of patients with treatment-resistant hypertension. *Ann Intern Med* 1990;112:270–277.

Nuesch R, Schroeder K, Dieterle T, et al.: Relation between insufficient response to antihypertensive treatment and poor compliance with treatment: A prospective case-control study. *BMJ* 2001;323:142–146.

Redon J, Campos C, Narciso ML, et al.: Prognostic value of ambulatory blood pressure monitoring in refractory hypertension. *Hypertension* 1998;31:712–718.

Setaro JF, Black HR: Refractory hypertension. *N Engl J Med* 1992;327:543–547.

Waeber B, Scherrer U, Petrillo A, et al.: Are some hypertensive patients overtreated? A prospective study of ambulatory blood pressure recording. *Lancet* 1987;2:732–734.

Yakovlevitch M, Black HR: Resistant hypertension in a tertiary care clinic. *Arch Intern Med* 1991;151:1786–1792.

#29 Special Patients: Children, the Elderly, and Blacks

HYPERTENSION IN CHILDREN

Hypertension in prepubertal children is rare, often symptomatic, and usually secondary to an identifiable cause. Hypertension in postpubertal children and adolescents is more common, usually asymptomatic, and more likely primary (or idiopathic). As BP measurements have been taken more frequently among young people, the presence of hypertension in as many as one percent of seemingly healthy adolescents has been recognized.

Small birth weight from intrauterine growth retardation is associated with higher BP in childhood and later life. A family history of hypertension, obesity, and high-normal BP recordings predict the future development of primary hypertension.

The suggested upper limits of normal BPs in children by age, gender, and height (50th percentile) from JNC-6 are:

Age (years)	Blood Pressure (mm Hg)	
	Girls	*Boys*
1	104/58	102/57
6	111/73	114/74
12	123/30	123/81
17	129/84	136/87

Prepubertal

The younger the patient with elevated BP, the more likely the hypertension represents a congenital problem. Such problems include:
- Coarctation of the aorta
- Renal hypoplasia

- Congenital adrenal hyperplasia
- Reflux nephropathy

Most advise a study of renal function and structure for every prepubertal child with hypertension without an obvious cause.

Postpubertal

The older the child, the more likely hypertension is primary. Obesity is a major factor, and weight reduction should be the first approach to therapy. Guidelines as to when to institute drug therapy and which drug should be used remain unsettled.

Some believe that evidence of LVH by echocardiography, present in a surprisingly high percentage of adolescents with presumably mild hypertension, is an indication for drug therapy. More information is needed, since some LVH may be a necessary response to the elevated afterload from increased vascular resistance.

HYPERTENSION IN THE ELDERLY

More than half of people older than age 65 will develop systolic hypertension, defined as BP above 140 mm Hg. People who develop significant diastolic hypertension after age 60 should be evaluated for renovascular disease. ISH reflects increasing atherosclerotic rigidity of large arteries and is the type of hypertension in two-thirds of the elderly with an elevated BP. Some who have very high cuff BP readings may have pseudohypertension from inability of the balloon to compress the calcified brachial artery.

The presence of ISH is associated with an increased risk of stroke, other cardiovascular

29.

diseases, and dementia, including Alzheimer's. Data from multiple clinical trials document the ability of antihypertensive therapy to lower such pressures and to remove such risks. The first, the Systolic Hypertension in the Elderly Program (SHEP), documented the benefits of therapy in reducing stroke, CHD, and CHF. Confirmation of the value of therapy came from the Working Party MRC trial in the elderly, and the more recent SYST-EUR and SYST-CHINA trials. In the first two studies, low doses of a diuretic or beta-blocker were used; in the SYST-EUR and SYST-CHINA trials, a long-acting dihydropyridine CCB was the primary drug.

Therapy (see Table 29.1)

Elderly people with systolic levels above 160 mm Hg or with diastolic levels above 95 mm Hg should be treated, since they are protected as well, if not better, than young patients by appropriate therapy. Lifestyle modification (described in Sections #9 and #10) should be tried, since elderly people respond particularly well to dietary reduction of sodium and regular exercise. Moreover, they may have more problems with drugs due to various age-related changes, including:

- Loss of baroreceptor responsiveness, increasing the propensity to postural hypotension (upright BPs should always be taken)
- Decrease in myocardial contractility
- Shrinkage of body fluid volume
- Decrease in renal excretory capacity
- Inability to remember doses and to open child-resistant bottles of drugs

The elderly are more likely to have other medical problems that may be aggravated by antihypertensive therapy (e.g., those with diabetes who take beta-blockers) or that involve use of medications that may interfere with hypertension therapy (e.g., NSAIDs with the action of diuretics, beta-blockers, ACEIs, or ARBs).

Choices of Drugs

Antihypertensive drugs should be given cautiously, with the initial goal of gradually and gently lowering SBPs to below 160 mm Hg and DBPs to below 95 mm Hg, with the eventual goal of 140 to 145 mm Hg systolic and 85 mm Hg diastolic.

The elderly will usually respond to any antihypertensive agent, but diuretics or CCBs may be the most effective and least bothersome. Additionally, they are the only classes that have been shown to reduce morbidity and mortality in the elderly. Cautions should be taken with every choice, accordingly:

- Diuretics—12.5 mg of HCT (preferably with a K^+ sparer) is an adequate starting dose so as not to decrease further a smaller fluid volume present in many.
- Central alpha-agonists may impair mental alertness.
- Beta-blockers may further reduce the ability to ambulate and exercise; some find that these interfere with sleep.
- Alpha-blockers are useful for those men with prostatism but should be given with a diuretic to prevent heart failure.
- Nondihydropyridine CCBs may worsen constipation (verapamil) or A-V conduction

problems (verapamil, diltiazem), but all types are usually effective.
- ACEI and ARBs usually work well if given with a diuretic with cautions about the presence of renovascular disease.

In those with ISH who often start with quite low diastolic pressure, caution is advised if, in lowering the elevated systolic pressure, the diastolic falls to below 65 mm Hg (Vokó et al. 1999).

HYPERTENSION IN BLACKS

Blacks have more hypertension and suffer more hypertension-related morbidity and mortality than nonblacks. Both genetic and environmental factors are responsible for the higher incidence of hypertension, including high levels of stress related to minority status and poverty. Restricted access to healthcare is involved in higher mortality from hypertension, since blacks are as well protected as are nonblacks with appropriate management. This population may also suffer more damage because of a lesser fall in BP during sleep.

A "stroke belt" in the southeastern United States and a much higher prevalence of ESRD are two manifestations of the higher incidence of hypertension and the lesser access to therapy provided to blacks in the United States.

Of the secondary forms of hypertension, renovascular disease is less common in blacks, whereas renal parenchymal damage is more common. The latter may mainly reflect more hypertension-induced nephrosclerosis.

Therapy

Treatment should emphasize dietary sodium restriction, since blacks tend to be more sodium sensitive, as reflected in generally lower levels of PRA.

Black patients tend to be equally or more responsive to diuretics, alpha-blockers, and CCBs but somewhat less responsive to beta-blockers and ACEIs than white patients. This lesser responsiveness to drugs that act by suppressing the renin-angiotensin mechanism is in keeping with usually lower PRA levels. With a diuretic to stimulate PRA, black patients respond well both to beta-blockers and ACEIs.

TABLE 29.1

Guidelines in Treating Hypertension in the Elderly

Check for postural and postprandial hypotension before starting.

Choose drugs that will help other concomitant conditions:

> For uncomplicated patients, a thiazide diuretic + K+ sparer.

> If a second agent is needed, a CCB.

> Beta-blockers are not appropriate unless an indication is present, e.g., coronary disease.

Start with small doses, titrating gradually.

Use longer-acting, once-daily formulations.

Avoid drug interactions, particularly from over-the-counter medications, e.g., NSAIDs.

Look for subtle drug-induced adverse effects, e.g. weakness, dizziness, depression, confusion.

Monitor home blood pressures to avoid over and under treatment.

Aim for the goal of SBP = 140-145, DBP = 80-85.

References

Children

Fernandes E, McCrindle BW: Diagnosis and treatment of hypertension in children and adolescents. *Can J Cardiol* 2000;16:801–811.

Flynn JT: Evaluation and management of hypertension in childhood. *Prog Pediatr Cardiol* 2001;12:177–188.

National High Blood Pressure Education Program Working Group: Update of the 1987 task force report on high blood pressure in children and adolescents. *Pediatrics* 1996;98:649–658.

Sinaiko AR, Donahue RP, Jacobs DR Jr., et al.: Relation of weight and rate of increase in weight during childhood adolescence to body size, blood pressure, fasting insulin, and lipids in young adults. *Circulation* 1999;99:1471–1476.

Elderly

Kivipelto M, Helkala E-L, Laakso MP, et al.: Midlife vascular risk factors and Alzheimer's disease in later life: Longitudinal, population based study. *BMJ* 2001;322:1447–1451.

Medical Research Council Working Party: MRC trial of treatment of hypertension in older adults: Principal results. *Br Med J* 1992;304:405–412.

Moore TJ, Conlin PR, Ard J, Svetkey LP: DASH (Dietary Approaches to Stop Hypertension) diet is effective treatment for stage 1 isolated systolic hypertension. *Hypertension* 2001;38:155–158.

Morgan TO, Anderson AIE, MacInnis RJ: ACE inhibitors, beta-blockers, calcium blockers, and diuretics for the control of systolic hypertension. *Am J Hypertens* 2001;14:241–247.

National High Blood Pressure Education Program Working Group: Report on hypertension in the elderly. *Hypertension* 1994;23:275–285.

SHEP Cooperative Research Group: Prevention of stroke by antihypertensive drug treatment in older persons with isolated systolic hypertension. *JAMA* 1991;265:3255–3264.

Tonkin AL: Postural hypotension. *Med J Australia* 1995;162: 436–438.

Vokó Z, Bots ML, Bots ML, Hofman A, et al. J-shaped relation between blood pressure and stroke in treated hypertensives. *Hypertension* 1999;34:1181–1185.

Wang J-G, Staessen JA: Antihypertensive drug therapy in older patients. *Curr Opin Nephrol Hypertens* 2001;10:263–269.

Blacks

Gillum RF: The epidemiology of cardiovascular disease in black Americans. *N Engl J Med* 1996;335:1597–1598.

James SA, Keenan NL, Strogatz DS, et al.: Socioeconomic status, John Henryism, and BP in black adults. *Am J Epidemiol* 1992;135:59–67.

Jamerson K, DeQuattro V: The impact of ethnicity on response to antihypertensive therapy. *Am J Med* 1996;22S–32S.

Sareli P, Radevski IV, Valtchanova ZP, et al.: Efficacy of different drug classes used to initiate antihypertensive treatment in black subjects. *Arch Intern Med* 2001;161:965–971.

Weir MR, Smith DHG, Neutel JM, Bedigian MP: Valsartan alone or with a diuretic or ACE inhibitor as treatment for African American hypertensives: Relation to salt intake. *Am J Hypertens* 2001;14:665–671.

NOTES

#30 Special Patients:
Diabetes, Dyslipidemia

Diabetes
Dyslipidemia

DIABETES

Diabetes mellitus and hypertension coexist more commonly than predicted by chance, perhaps three times more. Of the 10 percent of diabetics with the insulin-dependent form (IDDM) (type I), hypertension is seen in most of the 40 percent who develop nephropathy. In the 90 percent of diabetics with noninsulin-dependent (NIDDM) (type 2), almost all of whom are obese, hypertension is more common than among obese people without diabetes. The connection between hypertension, diabetes, and obesity is even stronger in those whose obesity is predominantly upper body, comprising the major components of the metabolic syndrome.

Complications

The diabetics in Framingham suffered almost twice as many strokes, three times more peripheral vascular disease and heart failure, and twice the number of coronary events than did nondiabetics. All these situations are increased further when hypertension accompanies diabetes. The microvascular complications, retinopathy in particular, also are increased by hypertension.

All diabetics should be carefully checked for microalbuminuria. If it is present, hypertension and diabetes should be carefully controlled to slow the progression of glomerulosclerosis.

All current guidelines recommend starting diabetics with BP > 130/85 on drug therapy. The goal of therapy is uncertain but, if feasible, BP should be lowered to below 130/80.

Antihypertensive Therapy

For the 90 percent of patients with NIDDM (type 2), the most useful therapy is weight reduction. If weight can be lost through diet and exercise, marked improvements in insulin resistance and BP can be accomplished.

If antihypertensive drugs are needed, they should be chosen carefully, with recognition of their many possible adverse effects (see Table 30.1). Most authorities recommend the use of either an ACEI or an ARB for initial therapy for diabetic hypertensives, with a diuretic as a second step. In the SHEP trial, low-dose diuretic-based therapy was as effective in preventing major cardiovascular events among older diabetic patients as it was in nondiabetics. CCBs are often needed as third drugs in order to achieve the goal of therapy.

ACEIs and ARBs are the best choice in the presence of diabetic nephropathy, slowing the progress of renal damage even when hypertension is not present. ACEIs have been utilized in trials of type 1 patients, ARBs in type 2 patients.

30.

Antidiabetic Agents

Metformin and thiazolidinedione derivatives such as troglitazone are being used to improve insulin sensitivity and help control diabetes. In short-term studies, they also lower BP.

DYSLIPIDEMIA

Three facts should be recognized in the relationship between hypertension and dyslipidemia. First, the two are more common together than expected by chance, likely from the contributions of obesity, diabetes, and alcohol abuse. Dyslipidemia adds further to the endothelial dysfunction typical of hypertension.

Second, some drugs used to treat hypertension may have either beneficial or deleterious effects on serum lipids (Table 30.1). Fortunately, these effects tend to be minimal and transient and in appropriate low doses not to interfere with the overall benefits of diuretic- or beta-blocker-based therapies on cardiovascular morbidity and mortality. Nonetheless, the special ability of alpha-blockers to reduce lipids adds to their attraction.

Third, treatment of dyslipidemia, in particular with statins, may have an independent effect of lowering BP. The current enthusiasm for the wider use of these drugs to treat dyslipidemia should only be heightened in patients with hypertension. Fortunately, no interferences with the actions of antihypertensive drugs or the effectiveness of statins occur when they are used simultaneously. Therefore, the way is clear for a much more intensive attack on the common combined threats of hypertension and dyslipidemia.

TABLE 30.1

Antihypertensive Drug Use with Diabetes or Dyslipidemia

DRUG CLASS	BENEFITS	PRECAUTIONS
Diuretics	Overcome volume expansion Improve efficacy of all other agents	May worsen insulin sensitivity May cause impotence, orthostatic hypotension, dyslipidemia
Alpha-blockers	Improve insulin sensitivity; Improve lipid status	May cause orthostatic hypotension (if used with diuretics)
Beta-blockers	Relieve angina Protective post-MI	May worsen insulin sensitivity Obscure and prolong hypoglycemic symptoms Raise serum triglycerides
Calcium channel blockers	No adverse effects on lipids or insulin sensitivity	Long-term effects on renal function uncertain
ACE inhibitors	Renal protection	Hyperkalemia particularly with hypoaldosteronism or K+ = sparing agents
A-II receptor blockers	Protective post-MI Relieve CHF	Loss of renal perfusion with renovascular disease

References

Diabetes

ACE Inhibitors in Diabetic Nephropathy Trialist Group. Should all patients with type 1 diabetes mellitus and microalbuminuria receive angiotensin-converting enzyme inhibitors? *Ann Intern Med* 2001;134:370–379.

Adler AI, Stratton IM, Neil HAW, et al.: Association of systolic blood pressure with macrovascular and microvascular complications of type 2 diabetes (UKPDS 36): Prospective observational study. *Br Med J* 2000;321:412–419.

Bakris GL, Williams M, Dworkin L, et al.: Preserving renal function in adults with hypertension and diabetes: A consensus approach. *Am J Kidney Dis* 2000;36:646–661.

Brenner BM, Cooper ME, de Zeeuw D, et al.: Effects of losartan on renal and cardiovascular outcomes in patients with type 2 diabetes and nephropathy. *N Engl J Med* 2001;345:861–869.

Curb JD, Pressel SL, Cutler JA, et al.: Effect of diuretic-based antihypertensive treatment on cardiovascular disease risk in older diabetic patients with isolated systolic hypertension. *JAMA* 1996;276:1886–1892.

Hovind P, Rossing P, Tarnow L, et al.: Progression of diabetic nephropathy. *Kidney Int* 2001;59:702–709.

Kaplan NM. Management of hypertension in patients with type 2 diabetes mellitus: Guidelines based on current evidence. *Ann Intern Med* 2001;135:1079–1083.

Kotchen TA: Attenuation of hypertension by insulin-sensitizing agents. *Hypertension* 1996;28:219–223.

Lewis EJ, Hunsicker LG, Clarke WR, et al.: Renoprotective effect of the angiotensin-receptor antagonist irbesartan in patients with nephropathy due to type 2 diabetes. *N Engl J Med* 2001;345:851–860.

Lithell HO: Hyperinsulinemia, insulin resistance, and the treatment of hypertension. *Am J Hypertens* 1996;9:150S–154S.

Mogensen CE, Neldam S, Tikkanen I, et al.: Combination therapy with candesartan and lisinopril was more effective than monotherapy in type 2 diabetes and hypertension. *Br Med J* 2000;321:1440–1444.

Dyslipidemia

Bonaa KH, Thelle DS: Association between blood pressure and serum lipids in a population: The TROMSO study. *Circulation* 1991;83:1305–1314.

Borghi C, Veronesi M, Prandin MG, et al.: Statins and blood pressure regulation. *Curr Hypertens Rep* 2001;3:281–288.

Grimm RH, Flack JM, Grandits GA, et al.: Long-term effects of plasma lipids on diet and drugs to treat hypertension. *JAMA* 1996;275:1549–1556.

Isomaa B, Almgren P, Tuomi T, et al.: Cardiovascular morbidity and mortality associated with the metabolic syndrome. *Diabetes Care* 2001;24:683–689.

Kasiske BL, Ma JZ, Kalil RSN, Louis TA: Effects of antihypertensive therapy on serum lipids. *Ann Intern Med* 1995;122:133–141.

#31 Special Patients: Cardiac Diseases/Cerebral Vascular Disease

Cardiac Diseases
Cerebral Vascular Disease

CARDIAC DISEASES

Coronary Artery Disease

The presence of angina is usually an indication for a beta-blocker. A CCB and nitrates may also be needed, and, on the basis of the HOPE trial, an ACEI will likely be given to most patients with or without hypertension. Hypertension that persists after an acute MI can logically be treated with a non-ISA beta-blocker and with a diuretic added if needed.

Hypertensive patients with atypical angina due to coronary spasm given beta-blockers may be susceptible to unopposed alpha-mediated vasoconstriction, although these agents' reduction in myocardial work usually leads to reduction in anginal attacks.

Patients early in the course of an acute MI may have a marked hypertensive response from pain- and stress-induced surges in catecholamine discharge. If BP remains very high despite relief of pain and anxiety, its careful reduction may be attempted under monitoring. Early use of beta-blockers has been advocated to reduce the extent of myocardial damage and may also be used to lower BP. IV nitroglycerin may be a better choice.

After the early period, continued use of oral beta-blockers has been shown to reduce recurrent MIs and mortality. Use of ACEIs post-MI has been shown to reduce the subsequent progression of myocardial dysfunction, CHF, and mortality. Some patients who were hypertensive before an MI have a marked fall in BP post-MI, which may be a bad prognostic sign if it reflects impaired myocardial function.

Reversal of Left Ventricular Hypertrophy

LVH is frequently present on echocardiography, even in patients with mild hypertension, and is a major independent risk factor for cardiovascular mortality. Most antihypertensive drugs have been shown to reverse LVH, ACEIs and CCBs somewhat better than diuretics and beta-blockers. Increasing evidence suggests that such reversal may be helpful, but it is not certain that the benefit goes beyond that obtained by reduction of BP.

Congestive Heart Failure

CHF is now classified as secondary either to LV systolic dysfunction, i.e., an ejection fraction less than 40%, or to LV diastolic dysfunction with increased filling pressure and a normal or even high ejection fraction. In systolic dysfunction, because neurohormonal activation as an attempt to maintain tissue perfusion plays such an important role, the value of ACEIs, other vasodilators, and beta-blockers has been recognized. A diuretic is given if there are evidences of fluid retention and spironolactone in Class III-IV CHF. An ARB may be substituted if the patient is intolerant of an ACEI.

There are no large outcome trials for diastolic dysfunction. Therapy is generally similar to systolic CHF with cautions to avoid excessive diuresis and tachycardia.

If a CCB is indicated, amlodipine or felodipine may be used, though no CCB has been shown to have a mortality benefit in CHF.

CEREBRAL VASCULAR DISEASE

Antihypertensive therapy has uniformly been found to reduce the occurrence of initial strokes and the mortality from them. Because hypertension is an independent risk factor for recurrent stroke, the control of hypertension offers the chance of preventing recurrences as well.

Acute Stroke

Caution is needed in the management of patients during the early course of stroke. These patients may have transient rises in BPs, presumably reflecting irritation of vasomotor centers or nonspecific responses to stress. Progression of acute stroke has been noted to be greater in patients with lower BPs on admission, so these transient rises may be needed to provide adequate cerebral blood flow (CBF). Therefore, immediate reduction of hypertension should only be attempted in patients with extremely high BPs (DBPs greater than 120 mm Hg), particularly in the presence of intracranial hemorrhage. Many antihypertensive agents (e.g., nitroprusside) increase intracranial pressure, whereas CCBs, ACEIs, and labetalol do not. If BP is lowered and brain function deteriorates, the pressure should be allowed to rise to ensure that blood flow is not being further reduced.

Chronic Therapy

CBF is kept very stable by adrenergically regulated changes in the caliber of cerebral arteries and arterioles. The range of cerebral autoregulation in normotensive people is roughly between 70/40 and 180/110 mm Hg. Levels below the lower limits induce a fall in CBF with signs and symptoms of hypotension; levels above the upper limits induce hyperperfusion of the brain that is responsible for hypertensive encephalopathy (see Section #33).

Patients with chronic hypertension have a shift to the right of the entire curve, reflecting the structural thickening of cerebral arteries. The range wherein autoregulation maintains normal CBF may then be between 140/90 and 210/130 mm Hg. Sudden lowering of BP to below 140/90 mm Hg, though certainly not to a truly hypotensive level, may nonetheless induce cerebral hypoperfusion and bring on postural dizziness, weakness, and faintness, explaining the frequent "washed-out" feelings that patients have when first using antihypertensive therapy that works too well. The better course is to go slowly, bringing BP down only 5 to 10 mm Hg at a time, and hopefully allowing CBF to be well maintained.

Fortunately, the range of cerebral autoregulation shifts back to the left with time, after persistent and gradual lowering of BP, presumably reflecting a decrease in the thickness of cerebral arteries. Thereby, lower levels of BPs, well into the truly normotensive range, may then be tolerated.

In the PROGRESS trial, recurrences of stroke were reduced by 43% with use of an ACEI (perindopril) and a diuretic (indapamide).

Caution is advised in lowering diastolic BP below 65 mm Hg in the elderly with ISH, as an increase in strokes has been noted in such patients.

References

Cardiac Diseases

Gomberg-Maitland M, Baran DA, Fuster V: Treatment of congestive heart failure. *Arch Intern Med* 2001;161:342–352.

Habib GB, Mann DL, Zoghbi WA: Normalization of cardiac structure and function after regression of cardiac hypertrophy. *Am Heart J* 1994;128:333–343.

Heart Outcomes Prevention Evaluation (HOPE) Study Investigators: Effects of an angiotensin-converting-enzyme inhibitor, ramipril, on cardiovascular events in high-risk patients. *N Engl J Med* 2000;342:145–153.

Hunick MGM, Goldman L, Tosteson ANA, et al.: The recent decline in mortality from coronary heart disease, 1980–1990. *JAMA* 1997;277:535–542.

Levy D, Larson MG, Vasan RS, et al.: The progression from hypertension to congestive heart failure. *JAMA* 1996;275:1557–1562.

Meredith PA: Implications of the links between hypertension and myocardial infarction for choice of drug therapy in patients with hypertension. *Am Heart J* 1996;132:222–228.

Pitt B, Poole-Wilson PA, Segal R, et al.: Effect of losartan compared with captopril on mortality in patients with symptomatic heart failure. *Lancet* 2000;355:1582–1587.

Pitt B, Zannad F, Remme WJ, et al.: The effect of spironolactone on morbidity and mortality in patients with severe heart failure. *N Engl J Med* 1999;341:709–717.

van Zwieten PA: The influence of antihypertensive drug treatment on the prevention and regression of left ventricular hypertrophy. *Cardiovasc Res* 2000;45:82–91.

Cerebral Vascular Disease

Blood Pressure Lowering Treatment Trialists' Collaboration: Effects of ACE inhibitors, calcium antagonists, and other blood-pressure-lowering drugs: Results of prospectively designed overviews of randomised trials. *Lancet* 2000;355:1955–1964.

Brott T, Bogousslavsky J: Treatment of acute ischemic stroke. *N Engl J Med* 2000;343:710–722.

Jorgensen HS, Nakayama H, Raaschou HO, Olsen TS: Effect of blood pressure and diabetes on stroke in progression. *Lancet* 1994;344:156–159.

Lai SM, Alter M, Friday G, Sobel E: A multifactorial analysis of risk factors for recurrence of ischemic stroke. *Stroke* 1994;25: 958–962.

PROGRESS Collaborative Group. Randomised trial of a perindopril-based blood-pressure-lowering regimen among 6105 individuals with previous stroke or transient ischaemic attack. *Lancet* 2001;358:1033–1041.

Strandgaard S, Paulson OB: Cerebrovascular consequences of hypertension. *Lancet* 1994;344:519–521.

Vokó Z, Bots ML, Hofman A, et al.: J-shaped relation between blood pressure and stroke in treated hypertensives. *Hypertension* 1999;34:1181–1185.

#32 Special Patients: Renal Insufficiency

As noted in Section #5, progressive renal insufficiency is a common consequence of sustained hypertension, particularly in blacks who often have more nephrosclerosis than whites with similar degrees of hypertension. Half of blacks who reach ESRD that requires dialysis therapy do so as a result of hypertension. A small proportion of whites develop ESRD from hypertension. Diabetic nephropathy is the most common and potentially preventable cause of ESRD; this, too, is more common in blacks, and its progress is accelerated by the usual coexistence of hypertension as renal function worsens.

Approximately 85 percent of patients with renal insufficiency will have hypertension, setting up the cycle of renal damage that causes hypertension that causes more renal damage. The process may involve sodium retention in most and the hypersecretion of renin in some. Patients with collagen vascular diseases may have rapidly accelerating hypertension because the intrarenal vascular disease activates renin release.

Ischemic nephropathy from bilateral renovascular disease should always be considered in patients with severe hypertension and progressive renal insufficiency.

In all forms of renal disease, proteinuria is usual and is, in itself, a cause of further renal damage.

Control of Fluid Volume
Control of sodium intake and excretion becomes increasingly important as renal function worsens. Dietary sodium restriction should help,

with the caution that overly rigorous restriction may cause those who have a fixed degree of sodium wastage to become volume depleted.

Diuretics are almost always needed. Thiazides generally work only if the GFR is above 30 ml/minute, reflected in a serum creatinine below 2.0 mg/dl. Those with more severe renal insufficiency will usually require a loop diuretic, although metolazone will work for many patients and requires only once-per-day dosage (see Section #14).

Other Therapy

In addition to adequate diuretic therapy, a number of other antihypertensive drugs may be used. For years, minoxidil has been effectively used in patients with severe hypertension related to renal insufficiency. Recently, ACEIs and ARBs have been used increasingly, since these drugs block the high concentrations of A-II at the efferent arterioles, preferentially dilating them, reducing intraglomerular pressure, and thereby slowing the progress of glomerular sclerosis.

Renal function may suddenly worsen in patients given ACEIs or ARBs if previous high levels of A-II were maintaining renal perfusion. This is most likely to occur in patients with bilateral renovascular disease or with a stenosis in the artery to a solitary kidney.

Overly aggressive falls in BP from any drug may, at least transiently, reduce renal blood flow and cause the serum creatinine to rise further. If the rise is not progressive or excessive, therapy should be continued, since successful long-term control of hypertension may lead to an improvement of renal function. Such improvement has

32.

been noted less commonly than hoped for, perhaps because not enough therapy has been provided to reduce BP to levels low enough to protect remaining nephrons, levels below 120/80 mm Hg. Often CCBs will be needed in addition to ACEIs/ARBs and diuretics to achieve adequate control.

The doses of various drugs that are excreted through the kidneys may need to be reduced as renal function deteriorates. ACEIs and ARBs may induce hyperkalemia, particularly when given with spironolactone or other K^+ sparers.

Other Therapies

Beyond tight control of hypertension, these have been shown to slow the progress of renal damage:

- In diabetics, control of glycemia
- Reduction of proteinuria by ACEI or ARB therapy
- Cessation of smoking
- Moderate restriction of dietary protein

Dialysis and Transplantation

When renal function nears the end, dialysis is usually necessary to bring BP under control. In some, the response is dramatic. Hypertension that was unmanageable on three or four medications may become easily controlled on small doses of one or two. In others, however, BP remains a problem, particularly on days between dialysis treatments. More frequent and prolonged hemodialyses or peritoneal dialyses will usually control even resistant hypertension.

Erythropoietin therapy may raise BP, largely as the consequence of the increased red cell mass.

The implantation of a normal kidney may relieve or cure hypertension even if it began as the primary (idiopathic) form. This suggests that primary hypertension may start from renal dysfunction. Unfortunately, a number of events in the posttransplant period may bring hypertension back. These include:

- Cyclosporine or tacrolimus therapy
- High doses of steroids
- Rejection
- Stenosis at the graft site

References

Agodoa LY, Appel L, Bakris GL, et al.: Effect of ramipril vs amlodipine on renal outcomes in hypertensive nephrosclerosis: A randomized controlled trial. *JAMA* 2001;285:2719–2728.

Bakris GL, Siomos M, Richardson DJ: ACE inhibition or angiotensin receptor blockade: Impact on potassium in renal failure. *Kidney Int* 2000;58:2084–2092.

Caetano ER, Zatz R, Saldanha LB, Praxedes JN: Hypertensive nephrosclerosis as a relevant cause of chronic renal failure. *Hypertension* 2001;38:171–176.

Coresh J, Wei GL, McQuillan G, et al.: Prevalence of high blood pressure and elevated serum creatinine level in the United States: Findings from the Third National Health and Nutrition Examination Survey (1988–1994). *Arch Intern Med* 2001;161:1207–1216.

Faguli RM, Reboldi G, Quintaliani G, et al.: Short daily hemodialysis: Blood pressure control and left ventricular mass reduction in hypertensive hemodialysis patients. *Am J Kidney Dis* 2001;38:371–376.

Klag MJ, Whelton PK, Randall BL, et al.: End-stage renal disease in African-American and white men. *JAMA* 1997;277:1293–1298.

Olyaei AJ, deMattos AM, Bennett WM: A practical guide to the management of hypertension in real transplant recipients. *Drugs* 1999;58:1011–1027.

Ruggenenti P, Schieppati A, Remuzzie G: Progression, remission, regression of chronic renal diseases. *Lancet* 2001;357:1601–1608.

Schrier RW, Estacio RO: The effect of angiotensin-converting enzyme inhibitors on the progression of nondiabetic renal disease: A pooled analysis of individual-patient data from 11 randomized, controlled trials. *Ann Intern Med* 2001;135:138–140.

Shankel SW, Johnson DC, Clark PS, et al.: Acute renal failure and glomerulopathy caused by nonsteroidal anti-inflammatory drugs. *Arch Intern Med* 1992;152:986–990.

Sturrock NDC, Lang CC, Struthers AD: Cyclosporine-induced hypertension precedes renal dysfunction and sodium retention in man. *J Hypertens* 1993;11:1209–1216.

Toto R: Angiotensin II subtype 1 receptor blockers and renal function. *Arch Intern Med* 2001;161:1492–1499.

Walls J: Relationship between proteinuria and progressive renal disease. *Am J Kidney Dis* 2001;37:S13–S16.

#33 Special Patients: Treatment of Hypertensive Crises

Emergencies vs Urgencies

Some patients with markedly elevated BPs may pose a therapeutic emergency. Their BPs may need to be reduced within minutes if there is immediate danger to the brain, heart, or large-vessel integrity or within hours if BP is so high as to pose an eventual threat to vascular and target-organ function. It is useful to segregate hypertensive emergencies from urgencies in order to select the best therapy:

Hypertensive emergencies include:
- Encephalopathy, including eclampsia
- Severe hypertension with progressing MI
- Intracranial hemorrhage
- Dissecting aortic aneurysm
- Hypertension immediately postoperative

Hypertensive urgencies include:
- Accelerated (Grade 3 fundi) or malignant (Grade 4) hypertension
- Diastolic levels above 140 mm Hg
- CHF
- Cerebral thrombosis
- Rapidly advancing renal ischemia, e.g., scleroderma crisis
- Intractable nose bleed
- Monoamine oxidase-tyramine interaction
- Sympathomimetic drug overdose
- Rebound from abrupt cessation of adrenergic-inhibiting drugs, e.g. clonidine

Drugs for Hypertensive Emergencies

When feasible, a hypertensive emergency patient should:

- Be admitted to an intensive-care unit
- Have an intra-arterial line inserted for constant monitoring of BP
- Be started on a parenteral agent (Table 33.1); in the past, this has usually been nitroprusside, but labetalol or nicardipine may be equally effective, easier to administer, and safer

Patients should have DBPs lowered to safe levels (usually below 120 mm Hg) to remove immediate danger but not so low as to reduce blood flow to vital organs. The safe diastolic level likely will be above 100 mm Hg.

If evidence of brain or heart ischemia develops, BPs can be allowed to rise to see if the lower pressure is responsible. If not, diastolic pressures should be kept between 100 and 120 mm Hg. Caution is needed to avoid reducing pressure too fast or too much.

Appropriate antihypertensive drugs should be started for more chronic therapy if patients can take oral medication. IV furosemide or torsemide may be needed to overcome the tendency toward fluid retention with successful lowering of BPs. However, diuretics may not be indicated initially and may actually be contraindicated if patients' fluid volumes are depleted from prior GI or renal losses.

Drugs for Hypertensive Urgencies

Patients in less tenuous conditions but with markedly high BPs have been successfully treated with numerous oral agents, including:
- Clonidine
- Captopril
- Nifedipine

33.

Liquid nifedipine, extracted from the capsule and either placed under the tongue or swallowed, has been widely used to bring very high BPs down quickly and smoothly. However, precipitous falls in BP may occur, rarely accompanied by acute cerebral or myocardial ischemia. Because there is no way to control response, the safer way is to use either parenteral drugs (as used for postoperative patients) or oral drugs that work within an hour (e.g., furosemide, captopril, propranolol, felodipine). The better way to manage patients with high BPs that pose no immediate danger is to remove any proximate causes (e.g., pain, distended bladder, etc.) and let them relax for 15 to 30 minutes. If BPs remain above 180/120 mm Hg, one of the semifast oral drugs could be used.

The goal of therapy is not simply to lower the high BP but to institute an effective regimen for long-term control that patients will take. This likely will require two or three oral drugs. These therapies can be started in small doses as soon as BPs have been brought down from dangerously high levels and control has been achieved and verified by checking patients one or two days after institution of therapy.

As with all hypertensive patients, particularly with those who have lesser elevations, these patients should have their BPs brought down in a steady and gradual manner so as not to reduce cerebral and other organ blood flow too much, thereby making patients dizzy, weak, or sedated.

Evaluation for Causes

Patients seen for hypertensive crises must have careful examinations to uncover underlying causes. Some causes may be obvious; however, renovascular disease is responsible in a significant number of patients. A renal angiogram should be done in all who do not have another obvious cause.

TABLE 33.1

Drugs for Hypertensive Crises

Drug	Dosage	Onset of Action	Adverse Effects[b]
Diuretics			
Furosemide	20-40 mg in 1-2 min, repeated and higher doses with renal insufficiency	5-15 min	Volume depletion, hypokalemia
Vasodilators			
Nitroprusside (Nipride, Nitropress)	0.25-10 µg/kg/min as i.v. infusion	Immediate	Nausea, vomiting, muscle twitching, sweating, thiocyanate and cyanide intoxication
Nitroglycerin (Nitro-bid IV)	5-100 µg/min as i.v. infusion	2-5 min	Headache, vomiting, methemoglobinemia, tolerance with prolonged use
Fenoldopam (Corlopam)	0.1-0.6 µg/kg/min as i.v. infusion	4-5 min	Reflex tachycardia, increased intraocular pressure, headache
Nicardipine (Cardene IV)	5-15 mg/h i.v.	5-10 min	Headache, nausea, flushing, tachycardia, local phlebitis
Hydralazine (Apresoline)	10-20 mg i.v. 10-10 mg i.m.	10-20 min 20-30 min	Tachycardia, flushing, headache, vomiting, aggravation of angina

Enalaprilat (Vasotec IV)	1.25-5 mg every 6	15 min	Precipitous fall in pressure in high-renin states; response variable
Adrenergic Inhibitors			
Phentolamine	5-15 mg i.v.	1-2 min	Tachycardia, flushing, headache
Esmolol (Brevibloc)	200-500 µg/kg/min for 4 min, then 50-300 µg/kg/min i.v.	1-2 min	Hypotension, nausea
Labetalol (Normodyne, Trandate)	20-80 mg i.v. bolus every 10 min 2 mg/min i.v. infusion	5-10 min	Vomiting, scalp tingling, burning in throat, dizziness, nausea, heart block, orthostatic hypotension

References

Adelman RD, Coppo R, Dillon MJ: The emergency management of severe hypertension. *Pediatr Nephrol* 2000;14: 422–427.

Grossman E, Messerli FH, Grodzicki T, Kowey P: Should a moratorium be placed on sublingual nifedipine capsules given for hypertensive emergencies and pseudoemergencies? *JAMA* 1996;276:1328–1331.

Lip GYH, Edmunds E, Hee FLLS, Blann AD, Beevers DG: A cross-sectional, diurnal, and follow-up study of platelet activation and endothelial dysfunction in malignant phase hypertension. *Am J Hypertens* 2001;14:823–828.

Neutel JM, Smith DHG, Wallin D, et al.: A comparison of intravenous nicardipine and sodium nitroprusside in the immediate treatment of severe hypertension. *Am J Hypertens* 1994;7: 623–628.

Strandgaard S, Paulson OB: Antihypertensive drugs and cerebral circulation. *Eur J Clin Invest* 1996;26:625–630.

Thach AM, Schultz PJ: Nonemergent hypertension. *Emerg Med Clin North Am* 1995;13:1009–1035.

Vaughn CJ, Delanty N: Hypertensive emergencies. *Lancet* 2000;356:411–418.

Ventura HO, Mehra MR, Messerli FH: Desperate diseases, desperate measures: Tackling malignant hypertension in the 1950s. *Am Heart J* 2001;142:197–203.

NOTES

#34 ABBREVIATIONS

ACEI	Angiotensin-converting enzyme inhibitor
ACTH	Adrenocorticotropic hormone
A-I	Angiotensin-I
A-II	Angiotensin-II
ALLHAT	Antihypertensive and Lipid-Lowering Treatment to Prevent Heart Attack Trial
ARB	Angiotensin-II receptor blocker
ARR	Aldosterone-to-renin ratio
BP	Blood pressure
A-V	Atrioventricular
CAD	Coronary artery disease
CBF	Cerebral blood flow
CCB	Calcium channel blocker
CHD	Coronary heart disease
CHF	Congestive heart failure
CNS	Central nervous system
CT	Computerized tomography
CVD	Cardiovascular disease
DBP	Diastolic blood pressure
ESRD	End-stage renal disease
ET-1	Endothelin-1
GFR	Glomerular filtration rate
GI	Gastrointestinal
HCT	Hydrochlorothiazide
HOPE	Heart Outcomes Prevention Evaluation
IDDM	Insulin-dependent diabetes mellitus
IM	Intramuscular
ISA	Intrinsic sympathomimetic activity
IV	Intravenous
JNC	Joint National Committee
KCl	Potassium chloride
LVH	Left ventricular hypertrophy
MEN	Multiple endocrine neoplasia
MI	Myocardial infarction
MRC	Medical Research Council
NaCl	Sodium chloride
NE	Norepinephrine
NEP	Neutral endopeptidase
NIDDM	Noninsulin-dependent diabetes mellitus
NSAID	Nonsteroidal anti-inflammatory drug
OC	Oral contraceptive
11-β-OHSD	11-β-Hydroxysteroid dehydrogenase
PRA	Plasma renin activity

PROGRESS	Perindopril Protection Against Recurrent Stroke Study
PIH	Pregnancy-induced hypertension
QOL	Quality of life
RCT	Randomized controlled trial
RVH	Renal vascular hypertension
SBP	Systolic blood pressure
SHEP	Systolic Hypertension in the Elderly Program
STONE	Shanghai Trial Of Nifedipine in the Elderly
SYST-CHINA	Systolic hypertension in China
SYST-EUR	Systolic hypertension in Europe
TOMHS	Treatment of Mild Hypertension Study
TSH	Thyroid-stimulating hormone
VA	Veterans Administration

34.